Stretching Exercises for Seniors

*Building Mobility and Flexibility
with Effective Workouts*

Table of Contents

Introduction

The older you get, the harder it becomes to stay active. Physical changes and constrictions can be challenging to deal with, so you need to adopt a healthy lifestyle as you navigate this stage in your life. This book is the key to increasing your flexibility, mobility, muscle range, and endurance. Reading it, you'll find beneficial information and practical techniques that will rejuvenate your body, release the pent-up tension you've accumulated over the years, and enhance the overall quality of your life.

This book is your gateway to exploring the transformative power of stretching. You will learn how to push your body's limits safely without risking injuries. It is your guide to controlled physical exercise whether you've been an athlete for your entire life or are only just discovering the power of stretching.

Very few people understand the aspirations and mental, physical, and emotional challenges seniors face when navigating their fitness and health journey. Hence, this book is tailored to your needs, ensuring that it is easy to understand and put into practice. You won't come across complicated, confusing jargon or demanding stretch and exercise routines.

This book promises step-by-step instructions and hands-on information everyone can follow.

The book delivers the importance and benefits of stretching for seniors and explores different stretching routines. You'll understand what each technique targets, determine if it's right for you, understand the potential risks, and learn to incorporate them into your routine safely. It gives an in-depth guide on how to prepare for stretching, examples of warm-up exercises, and the equipment you'll need.

You'll learn to execute upper body stretches properly and find instructions on how to release built-up stress in your neck, shoulders, arms, wrists, and upper back. You'll also discover a variety of exercises targeting your lower body. The book offers gentle full-body stretches that are yoga- and tai-chi-inspired.

One of the best things about this book is that it factors in age-related conditions. For instance, you'll find stretches to aid with arthritis relief, osteoporosis prevention, and chronic pain management. You will explore how you can progress with stretching and overcome the challenges that might arise throughout your fitness journey.

Reading this book, you learn to avoid common stretching mistakes and injuries. You will discover helpful nutrition, stress-reduction, and hydration tips to help improve your overall lifestyle and well-being.

Chapter 1: Understanding Stretching

While growing older and experiencing physical changes is a normal part of life, adapting to and embracing the golden years is easier said than done. You must take several measures to counter, or at least minimize, the effects of aging and maintain a good quality of life. Believe it or not, stretching can make a world of difference.

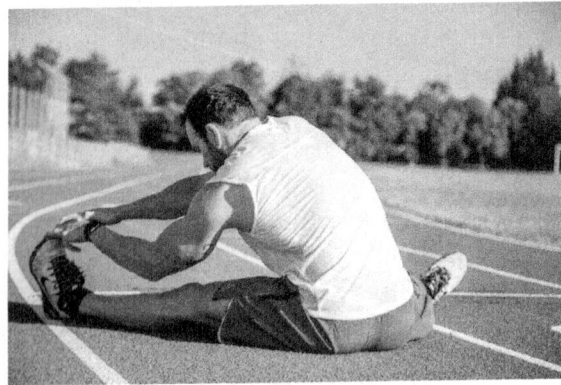

1. *Regular stretching can boost your mental, emotional, and physical health and is great for overcoming the challenges that come with the natural aging process. Source: https://unsplash.com/photos/man-in-white-sleeveless-top-WX7FSaiYxK8*

Regular stretching can boost your mental, emotional, and physical health and is great for overcoming the challenges that come with the natural aging process. Reading this chapter, you will learn about the different stretching exercises, their benefits and risks, and how to perform them properly. You'll understand how stretching impacts the aging process and why it is important for seniors.

The Mental and Physical Effects of Aging

Bodies naturally undergo a series of physical changes affecting your capabilities, quality of life, and general health as you age. Besides the medical conditions that arise, decreased flexibility, muscle mass, strength, balance, bone density, and balance are among the most common effects. As your flexibility and mobility declines, your ability to perform your daily activities becomes hindered. A lack of balance and coordination also puts you at greater risk of injuries, falls, and accidents.

Leading a sedentary lifestyle exacerbates the obstacles of everyday life for everyone, not just older adults. Anyone who barely engages in physical activities is likely to experience a decline in their range of movement, flexibility, strength, and overall well-being. Therefore, you must proactively counter the effects of aging and make an effort to maintain your muscle mass and cardiovascular fitness. Staying active can boost your energy and increase drive and motivation, which boosts your health and lowers your risk of developing mental health conditions like depression.

Stretching Can Slow Down Aging

No matter how old you are, you can slow down the aging process if you stretch regularly. A lack of flexibility results in shorter muscles, which leads to a smaller range of motion and poor posture. Being flexible is essential for doing daily tasks and chores easily.

While not being able to reach a higher shelf in your cupboard or struggling to pick up something from the floor might seem like small inconveniences, your physical capabilities will continue to decline if you don't start moving your body beneficially.

If you don't proactively counter the consequences of the golden age, you will further strain and tighten your joints, making it even harder to move freely. A lack of physical exercise can lead to an early onset of aging. Someone in their 40s can have the joints of a 60-year-old if they lead a sedentary lifestyle And, conversely, with regular exercise, a 60-year-old can have the joints of a 40-year-old.

If you're new to your fitness and stretching journey, consult a physical therapist to create a stretching program tailored to your needs. While this book is a good starting point for navigating the world of stretching and physical well-being, you should consider your current muscle and joint health, endurance, and any medical conditions when creating a stretch routine. Working with a professional will help you prevent injuries and ensure you obtain your desired results.

Create a stretching routine that targets various muscles simultaneously. You should work on strengthening and releasing tension in your neck, shoulders, upper and lower back, hip flexors, calves, and other areas of the body. For the best results, you should stretch every day or at least 3 times a week. If you stretch daily, you don't have to maintain the same intensity, duration, and stretching exercise. Change things up to target different muscle groups, achieve various fitness goals, and avoid getting bored.

Types of Stretching

Static Stretching

This is the most common form of stretching. Static stretching requires holding a position that exercises the targeted muscle group for at least 30 seconds. Slowly and gently move into your stretch position without making any sudden movements. Stretch until you feel mild tension building up in your muscles. You should feel a moderate stretch in the targeted area but not pain. Hold your position for 30 seconds and work on building your endurance daily until you reach 1 minute for a deeper stretch.

The two types of this exercise are active and passive stretching. The former requires actively engaging your muscles without the help of an external force. Passive stretching requires the assistance of an external force, like a prop or another person. Use equipment like a stretching strap, or ask someone to apply a controlled and gentle force to increase the intensity of the stretch and help you build mild muscle tension. Don't actively engage with the exercise.

Dynamic Stretching

Instead of holding one position, dynamic stretching is more like a stretch flow. You're required to do a series of continuous movements inspired by a particular sport or exercise's movements. This stretching can improve mobility and flexibility and help improve your performance in the sport you're mimicking.

Dynamic stretching prepares the body and muscles for optimal performance, increases blood flow, and helps with neuromuscular activation. It is a well-rounded exercise, as it also mentally prepares you for the physical and mental demands of the actual sport or exercise. For example, if someone is sprinting for a sport, they might practice extra-long strides. If they play golf, their stretch flow might include arm circles, leg swings, hip rotations, and torso twists.

Ballistic Stretching

This is considered dynamic stretching and requires incorporating a bouncing or pulsing motion to a specific muscle group throughout your stretch flow. Instead of building muscle tension in a fixed position, as you would do in a static stretch, ballistic stretching requires engaging your joints to create a bouncing motion.

Quick, continuous pulsing motions can trigger a stretch reflex in the target muscle groups, encouraging them to contract. While it is an effective stretching type, it's not as safe and gentle as other stretching techniques. You should be very careful and controlled with each movement to avoid getting injured or straining your muscles. It's best to consult a physical therapist for guidance on how to incorporate ballistic and other stretches into your routine safely.

Active Isolated Stretching

This stretching requires holding a stretch that targets a specific muscle group for only 2 seconds for several isolated bursts. When performing this stretch technique, you should gradually push and intensify the stretch a little further with each repetition, making each movement more effective. Active Isolation Stretching, or AIS is the strength-training and endurance-building routine for stretching. Start with a few repetitions and sets until you get the hang of your stretch routine.

Doing your stretches in short bursts allows you to avoid triggering the stretch response and reduces your risk of injury.

Gradually controlling your movements lengthens your targeted muscles. Repeating the movements builds your muscles' flexibility and increases your range of motion without leading to discomfort.

Myofascial Release

This stretching technique requires using equipment like stretch rollers to relieve tension and increase your fascia's flexibility. Start by doing each movement for 30 seconds and gradually increase until you're able to complete 1 minute. It is among the most effective exercises for releasing tension and improving mobility. Be mindful of your pain tolerance when applying pressure to the targeted muscles during your stretch. To avoid injury, don't try to withstand more than you can bear.

Doing a myofascial release involves using a foam roller to make continuous, controlled back-and-forth movements over the targeted body area. The pressure applied using the foam roller should be enough to feel a mild stretch and release tension in your muscles, but not so much that it hurts. Each person has different pressure adjustments, depending on their comfort level and pain tolerance.

Isometric Stretching

This stretching exercise is more suitable for individuals who have always been active throughout their lives. However, it also must be done with caution and under the supervision of a professional, as it is meant to help you achieve a significantly wider range of motion and enhance your overall strength in stretching exercises.

It requires stretching a certain muscle group and using a prop, like a chair, wall, or floor, to apply resistance without causing the body part (for example, the arm or leg) to bend.

An example of isometric stretching would be to extend your arm in front of you and place your palms flat on the wall at shoulder height. Then, push, without bending your elbows, as if you want to move the wall. You maintain this position for 15 to 30 seconds while breathing normally. Rest for a few seconds and repeat the exercise again, gradually increasing the intensity of the pressure over time. Another example would be stretching a single leg on a chair and trying to press your heel so your foot is flat against the back of the chair.

Proprioceptive Neuromuscular Facilitation Stretching

PNF, or Proprioceptive Neuromuscular Facilitation stretching, is a technique that combines static stretching with isometric contractions. It means that you constantly alternate between 15 to 30 seconds of stretching and 10 to 15 minutes of contractions. This exercise enhances flexibility and range of motion but must be conducted carefully. Like Ballistic Stretching, PNF can lead to muscle or joint injuries if done incorrectly.

Hold-relax is among the easiest PNF stretching techniques. Start with a stretch that targets a specific muscle group and hold it for a few seconds. Then, contract the same muscle group and hold your position for a few seconds. This technique helps lengthen the length of time for which you can hold a stretch.

The Importance of Stretching for Seniors

It Relieves Lower Back Pain and Alleviates the Symptoms of Arthritis

Often, older adults who struggle with lower back pain suffer from osteoarthritis. This arthritis is due to the gradual breakdown of cartilage, resulting in lower back pain. The condition also affects other areas, such as the neck, hips, and knees. Around 33.6% of seniors, 65 years old and above, are affected by osteoarthritis.

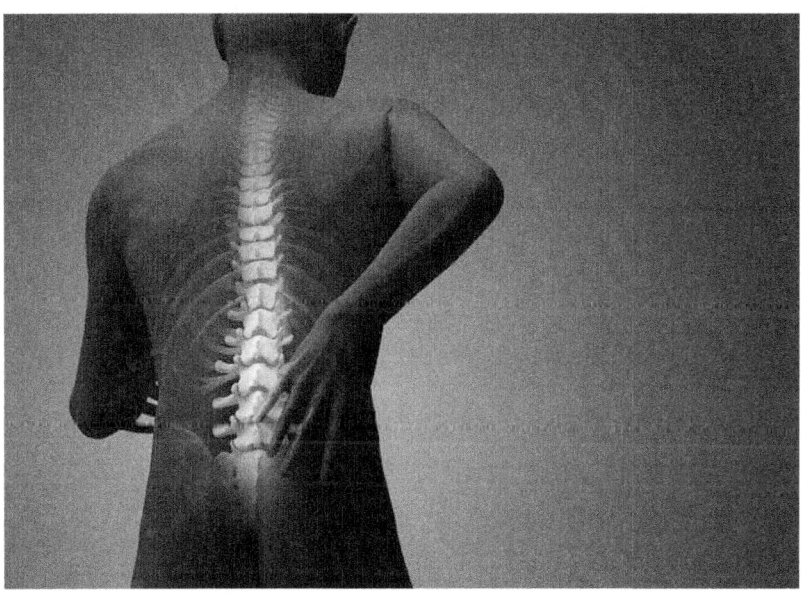

2. *Often, older adults who struggle with lower back pain suffer from osteoarthritis. Source: https://pixabay.com/illustrations/man-lower-back-pain-back-pain-8362961/*

Spinal stenosis is another condition older adults with lower back pain might struggle with. It is characterized by a narrowing of the bone channel, which compresses the spinal nerves or cords and results in this pain. In addition to back aches, the affected individuals may experience symptoms like numbness and tingling.

While both conditions are usually a natural part of the aging process and can't be entirely prevented, incorporating stretches into your routine will lead to better pain and symptom management. At first, it can be difficult to stretch your muscles and move your joints. However, it becomes easier, and you'll feel more comfortable with practice. Use a heat pack before you start stretching and an ice pack afterward to reduce muscle stiffness and joint swelling. You could consider asking someone to help and guide you, at least until you get the hang of it.

It Lowers the Risk of Falling

As you grow older, your muscle mass, bone density, and strength all decline, which results in a higher risk of falling. However, stretching can help you counter these risks, as it increases your range of motion, improves your balance, strengthens your core muscles, and enhances your posture and flexibility.

Stretching Reduces Stiffness in Arteries

Arteries are supposed to maintain their elasticity, even as you age. However, seniors often develop stiffness in their arteries due to a lack of physical activity. Stretching can improve your overall flexibility and mobility and release body tension, preventing arterial stiffness.

It Decreases Pain

Seniors who stretch regularly experience a decrease in several body aches and report better pain management. Stretching helps you feel better because it increases blood flow, releases joint tension and stiffness, improves muscle and joint function, and releases endorphins.

Stretching Supports Walking and Other Forms of Exercise

Stretching positively impacts your pelvis' tilt and increases your range of motion, which can lengthen your strides and make them quicker. Stretching also enhances strength and endurance, which support other forms of exercise.

Stretching Lowers the Risk of Injury

Stretching can help you lower the risk of injury because it enhances muscle flexibility. A lack of muscle flexibility restricts and stiffens your joints, preventing them from maintaining their normal range of motion and affecting mobility. Generally, stiffness makes you more likely to overstretch and strain your muscles. This is why it's best to start with easy movements and maintain them for a few seconds. Be careful not to overextend yourself until you feel ready to elevate your stretch routine.

It Improves Posture

The water content in your ligaments, tendons, and other connective tissue decreases as you age, reducing their elasticity and making you less flexible. This results in stiffness in the connective tissue around your chest and shoulders, making you more likely to slouch, have a rounded upper back and shoulders, and develop poor posture. Stretching loosens up your connective tissues and grants you a greater range of motion, allowing you to keep your shoulders and upper back in proper stance.

It Facilitates Your Daily Activities

Daily activities, like lifting grocery bags, tying your shoes, and climbing the stairs, can become harder to do as you age. Not only can this get in the way of your routine and decrease your overall quality of life, but it can also result in frustration and low self-esteem. Fortunately, stretching can help you overcome these challenges and make your life much easier.

It's Great for Relaxation

Many stretch techniques encourage you to breathe deeply and practice mindfulness, which can relieve stress and lower anxiety. It also unties the knots in your muscles as it gently lengthens and stretches them, relieving muscle stiffness and discomfort.

Safety Considerations

Know Your Limits and Prioritize Your Safety

You need to consider several things to avoid hurting yourself as you embark on your fitness journey. Your safety and well-being should be your topmost priority when stretching. While it's good to challenge yourself, going far beyond your limits is a form of self-sabotage. The best progress is slow, gradual, and steady. It should be sustainable so you can achieve the best results.

Consider Your Balance

If you struggle with poor balance, you should start with exercises that can be performed in lying or seated positions. Supporting your body while stretching, especially if you're not well-balanced, can be challenging. Doing standing exercises when you lack balance can lead to falls and accidents. However, you should consider switching to seated or lying stretch positions if you feel unsteady or tired throughout your routine, even if you have no problem with balance.

With enough practice, your muscles will strengthen and become more flexible, allowing you to try standing stretch positions. Once you get used to moving your body this way, you should gradually introduce standing exercises into your stretch routine, as they are essential for improving balance. Start with easy stretches and use a prop, like a chair, for support. Be sure to maintain proper form and technique to reap the most rewards and avoid accidentally hurting yourself. It also helps to keep your feet apart to find your gravity center as you do standing exercises.

Declutter the Space

Ensure you have enough free space to stretch before starting your routine. Declutter the area and push potential obstacles out of your way to avoid accidentally bumping into or falling over an object. Focus on controlling your position and moving slowly and cautiously.

Follow a Warm-Up Routine

Following a warm-up routine before you start stretching will improve your blood flow and increase your range of motion in a short period of time, making you more flexible and less prone to injury as you stretch or exercise. Warm-up routines are often dynamic and take 5 to 10 minutes to complete.

End with Static Stretching

It's generally preferred to end your workout with static stretches since they're most effective when your muscles are warm. Your temperature and blood flow will increase throughout the workout, making the muscles more responsive to stretching. Performing static stretching at the end of your routine allows you to reap the most benefits from the movement and lower your risk of injury.

Doing static stretches while your muscles are warm and receptive will gradually make you more flexible and increase the range of motion of your muscles and joints. This stretching helps your muscles lengthen and relax after you've worked out. It is also considered part of the cool-down process, as it allows your breathing and heartbeats to return to their resting rates.

Consider the Weather

You should consider alternating between outdoor and indoor stretching sessions depending on the weather and humidity, as your tolerance to heat and humidity generally decreases as you grow older. Try to do your stretching routine early in the morning or late in the afternoon when the temperatures are lower. Stretching in the morning will allow you to start your day on a positive, relaxed note. If you're exercising indoors, make sure that the space is well-ventilated and the temperature is easily controlled.

Hydrate Properly and Dress Accordingly

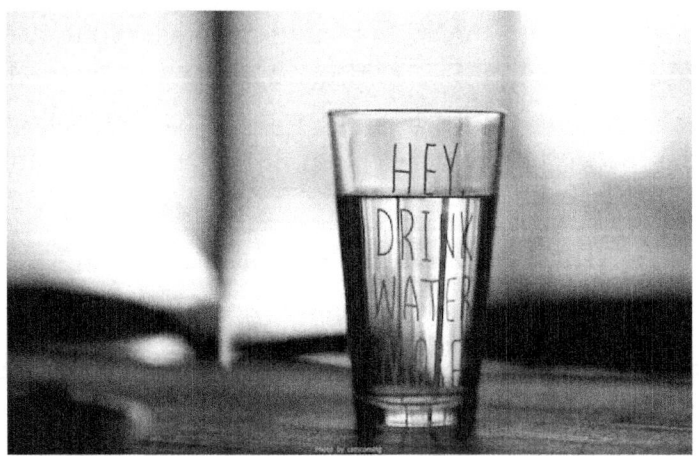

3. Always drink a lot of water before, during, and after your stretching session to stay well-hydrated. Source: https://www.pexels.com/photo/clear-drinking-glass-1633940/

Always drink a lot of water before, during, and after your stretching session to stay well-hydrated. Opt for lightweight and breathable clothes to dry the sweat and help your body stay cool. Additionally, choose loose-fitting and light-colored garments during the summer.

Practice Post-Exercise Hygiene, Get Good Quality Sleep, and Eat a Balanced Diet

Shower or wash up after you exercise to cool down and remove the sweat to help regulate your body temperature and avoid developing skin-related conditions. Get at least 7 hours of good quality sleep at night, and eat a well-balanced diet to help your muscles recover and support your immune system. Make sure your diet is rich in lean proteins, fruits, and vegetables to provide you with the necessary nutrients. Also, get periodic health checkups to improve your overall health and manage conditions that may be affected by heat or physical activity.

Look out for Signs of Fatigue

Look out for signs of fatigue or health issues while stretching, such as excessive sweating, weakness, dizziness, or loss of balance, and take immediate action. End your workout, relocate to a cooler room, hydrate, and reach out to a doctor if necessary.

When constructing a stretch or workout routine, you must be aware of your physical capabilities and underlying mental health conditions to tailor a plan to your needs. While this book is a great starting point for stretching, working with a professional to modify your stretch routine to lower your risk of injury is advisable. You should always prioritize safety, monitor your safety, and regularly check up on your overall well-being.

Chapter 2: Preparing for Stretching

Now that you understand stretching and its significance, you are ready for the next step. You probably think you should start stretching right away, well, not just yet. You should do a few things first to prepare for stretching. Start with some warm-up exercises to prevent injuries and get the most out of your workout. You should also set up a stretching space to practice freely with no distractions. You also can't start stretching without the proper equipment. So, what will you need? Well, you will find all this information in this chapter.

Warm-Up Exercises

Warm-up exercises are physical activities that prepare you mentally and physically for the demands of workouts or sports. These exercises strengthen your tendons, muscles, ligaments, and joints and elevate your heart rate so you are ready for practice.

Warm-up exercises fall into three categories: mobility, flexibility, and aerobics.

- Aerobics involves moving your large muscles repetitively and in continuous motion, like light jogging, jumping jacks, and walking, to improve circulation and increase your heart rate.

- Flexibility techniques stretch the soft tissues so you can move easily during exercises.

- Mobility exercises strengthen the joints so you can practice different workouts. Perform warm-ups for about 5 or 15 minutes before stretching.

Benefits of Warm-Up Exercises

- Reduces the risk of injury.

- Improves exercise performance.

- Engages your brain with your body.

- Loosens the joints.

- Easier muscle contraction.

- Releases more oxygen in the blood.

- Increases blood supply to the muscles.

- Raises the body's temperature.

- Slowly increases heart rate to reduce stress on the heart.

- Motivates you to exercise.

- Reduces muscle tension.

- Boosts your metabolism.

- Increases flexibility.

Check these warm-up exercises and practice one or more before stretching.

Arm Swinging

This is a simple and effective exercise that prepares you for stretching. It will boost your energy, reduce muscle tension, and keep your mind and body active. You can practice it while sitting, standing, or walking.

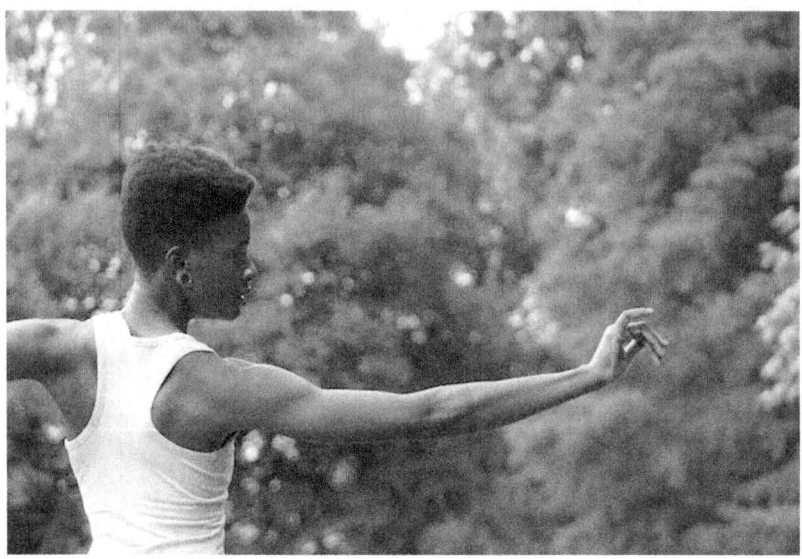

4. Arm swinging will boost your energy, reduce muscle tension, and keep your mind and body active. Source: https://www.pexels.com/photo/a-woman-stretching-her-arms-11038522/

Instructions:

1. Stand upright with your feet slightly apart.

2. Lift your arms to shoulder height.

3. Swing both arms simultaneously to the front and let them cross in front of your chest.

4. Then, swing them wide and behind.

Shoulder Circles

This exercise protects you against strains and prepares your arms for stretching exercises. It also strengthens your arm muscles to improve stability and balance and reduce the risk of injury.

Instructions:

1. Sit on a comfortable chair in an upright position.

2. Place your arms by your side, then put your fingertips on your shoulders.

3. Move your arms clockwise in circular motions 15 times.

4. Then, move your arms anti-clockwise 15 times.

Air Squats

Air squats can be demanding, but they are worth it. Many seniors struggle with knee problems that prevent them from practicing physical activity. If you have knee spasms or cramps every time you work out, you will usually give up and stop exercising. Luckily, warm-ups like air squats can protect you against knee issues. It also maintains your stamina and core strength.

Instructions:

1. Spread your feet shoulder-width apart and pull your hips down as if you are about to sit on a chair (don't use a chair for this workout).

2. Pull your body back up at a moderate pace.

3. Repeat these steps for five minutes.

Bicep Curls

You can practice this exercise wherever you want. You only need resistance bands. Choose X-heavy or X-light depending on your strengths, past experiences, and resistance level.

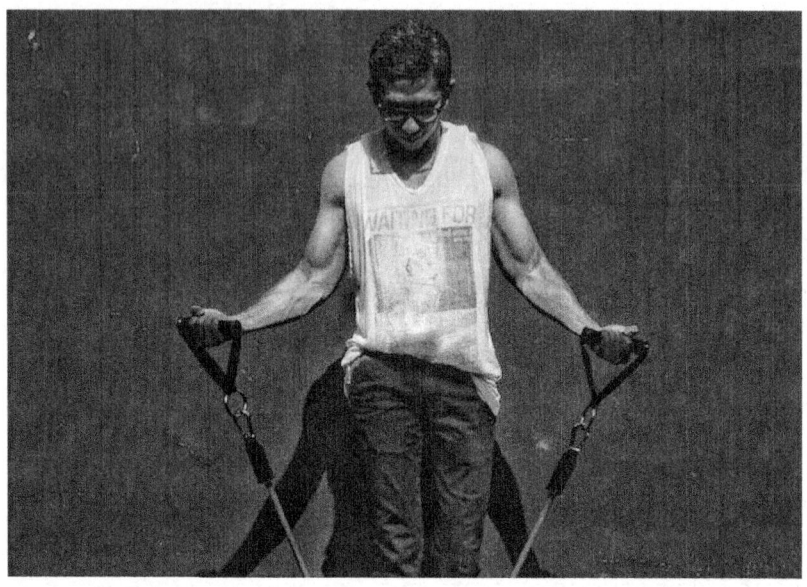

5. You can practice bicep curls wherever you want. Source: https://www.pexels.com/photo/a-man-using-a-resistance-band-6667512/

Instructions:

1. Place your feet slightly apart on the resistance band while standing up straight.

2. Grasp the band's grips with your arms extended straight forward and your palms facing upward.

3. Have your hands curled up against your shoulders.

4. As you slowly lower the resistance band, keep your elbows by your sides. In place of the bands, you can also use lightweight dumbbells.

Hula Hoops for the Hips

If you are looking for a fun and enjoyable warm-up, this is the one for you. You can use a hula hoop, but the exercise will work just as well without one. It reduces stress, improves your physical fitness, and gets the adrenaline in your body pumping. This exercise is very easy. Simply rotate your hips with a hula hoop. If you don't have one, just pretend you are practicing with one.

Shoulder Rolls

This warm-up exercise engages your muscles and shoulders.

Instructions:

1. Sit up straight and plant both of your feet firmly on the ground.

2. After shrugging, spin your shoulders back, down, forward, and back up in a circle.

3. After you get to the top, switch around the motions. Move your shoulders front, back, down, and finally upward.

4. Do this 10 times in each direction.

Ankle Circles

Ankle circles are a lot simpler than they sound. It is a great warm-up exercise for stretches that require moving your feet. It relaxes your foot muscles and prevents spasms, sprains, cramps, and injuries. Simply rotate your feet clockwise, then anti-clockwise in circles.

Triceps Extensions

Instructions:

1. Take a seat in a cozy chair.

2. With your shoulders back and your abs taut, grab a hand weight with your right hand and raise it to reach behind your head.

3. Use your left hand to brace your upper arm.

4. Raise and then lower your right arm above your head.

Brisk Walking

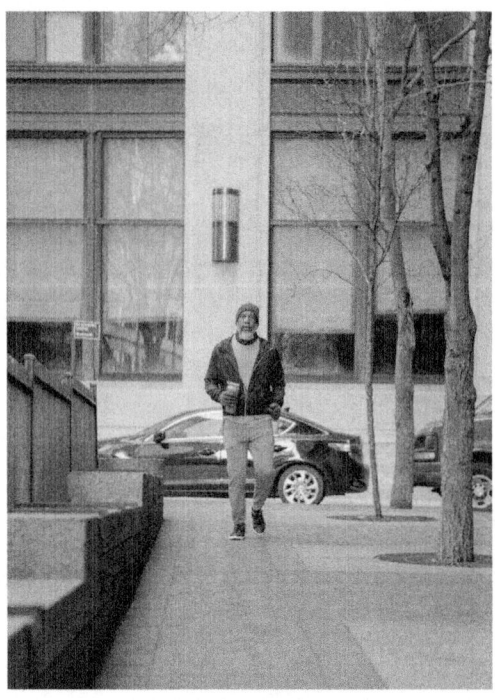

6. *Brisk walking is more effective and has more health benefits than walking at a moderate pace. Source: https://www.pexels.com/photo/trendy-senior-black-man-walking-along-sidewalk-7869652/*

This exercise is also called power walking and is simply walking faster than normal. It is more effective and has more health benefits than walking at a moderate pace. Since heart problems are common at this stage of your life, you need to focus on exercises that keep you healthy and build stamina. Although regular walking is one of the most common warm-up exercises, brisk walking is preferable since it reduces stress on the heart and elevates your heart rate.

Toe Taps

This warm-up exercise improves mobility and strengthens your muscles and calves.

Instructions:

1. Sit in an upright position with your feet hip-width apart and placed firmly on the ground.

2. Bend your toes upward, then downward.

Knee Lifts

Knee lifts increase your quad strength, which impacts your whole body and improves performance.

Instructions:

1. Sit in an upright position with your feet shoulder-width apart and flat and lift your left knee to your chest, then lower it so your foot touches the ground. Repeat this step 10 times.

2. Repeat the previous step with your right knee 10 times.

3. If you want to make this exercise harder and challenge yourself, pause for five seconds each time you lift your knee.

Sit-to-Stands

This exercise improves your balance and increases muscle strength.

Instructions:

1. Sit up straight on a comfortable chair with your feet flat on the floor, toes pointed forward, and have your abs tightened.

2. Place both hands on your thighs.

3. Slowly stretch both your arms forward, then stand up while keeping the same posture.

4. You should experience tension in the legs and hips.

5. Sit again while maintaining the same posture. Repeat ten times.

Sit and Reach

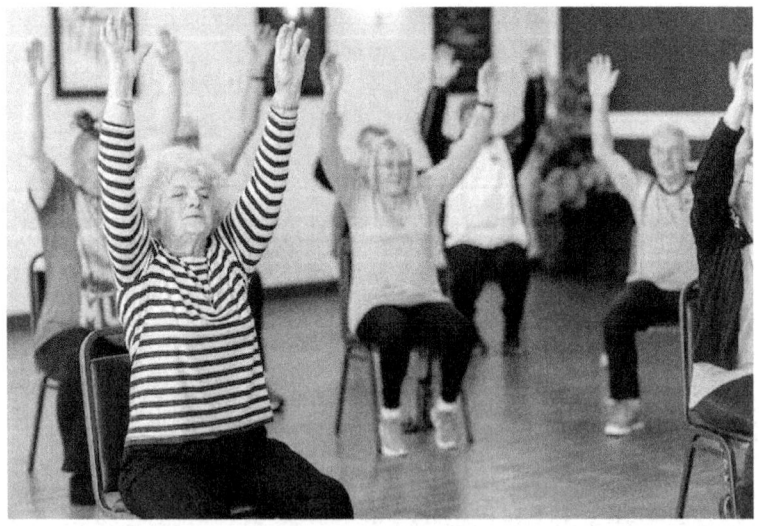

7.   Try reaching as high as you can. Source:
https://www.pexels.com/photo/seniors-exercising-11674389/

Instructions:

1. Sit in an upright position with your knees close together and feet flat on the floor.

2. Extend your right arm toward the ceiling and stretch the upper part of your body.

3. Lift your head up to stretch your shoulders and neck.

4. Stay in this position for ten seconds.

5. Repeat the steps with your other arm.

Seated Tap Dance

Instructions:

1. Sit on a comfortable chair with your feet on the floor slightly apart, toes lightly touching the ground, and knees slightly bent.

2. Gently touch the floor with your heel as you extend your right leg forward without raising it off the ground.

3. Point your toes forward, keep your legs extended, and tap them on the ground.

4. Extend your foot and tap your heel once more.

5. Repeat the previous steps with your left foot.

6. Since this is your first time, perform this exercise for three minutes. Set a timer and increase the timer each time.

Chair Running

Instructions:

1. Sit on a chair and extend your legs off the ground.

2. Place your arms by your sides and slightly bend your elbows.

3. Adjust your posture so that your shoulders and back hardly make contact with the chair's back.

4. Then, lift your feet as if you are riding a bike, extend your left knee, and pull your right knee toward you.

5. Move your legs as if you are running.

6. For balance, grip the sides of your chair.

Skater Switch

Instructions:

1. Sit on the edge of your seat.

2. Raise your left heel off the ground, keeping your toes on the floor.

3. With your toes pointing to the other side, extend your right leg straight out in front of you.

4. Lean your body forward and extend both arms in front of you.

5. Raise your left arm fully behind your body and use your right arm to reach the insole of your left foot.

6. Next, sit up straight and extend your arms in front of you.

7. Do this repeatedly, switching sides.

Seated Jumping Jacks

This exercise boosts coordination and mobility and promotes heart and bone health.

Instructions:

1. Sit up straight on the edge of your chair and bring your knees and feet together. The feet should be flat on the floor.

2. Start with your arms by your sides, elevate them to the side like a jumping jack, and then lower them back down.

3. Repeat 20 times.

4. Start at a slow pace, gradually increasing it.

Captain's Chair #1

This exercise increases your core muscles and abdominal' strength.

Use a strong chair for this technique.

Instructions:

1. Sit up straight and hold onto the edges of your chair. Choose a chair without arms for this exercise.

2. Gently lift your feet off the ground and move your knees to your chest.

3. Squeeze your top abs, then lower your feet to the ground.

4. If this exercise makes you uncomfortable, only lift your feet a couple of inches off the ground.

Captain's Chair #2

This is the perfect warm-up exercise for your core and arms.

Instructions:

1. Stand and face a chair. You should be standing close to the chair.

2. Bend over and put your palms on each armrest of the chair.

3. Then, shift your legs backward until your back is straightened.

4. Stay in this position for 30 seconds.

Wrist Rotation

This simple exercise increases blood flow in your wrists, so you are prepared for stretching and other exercises.

Instructions:

1. Sit up straight on a comfortable chair.

2. Extend your arms to the front with your palms facing downward.

3. Clench both fists, then open and close them four times,

4. Then, clasp your fingers together.

5. Rotate your wrists in all directions 10 times.

6. Do this exercise for one minute.

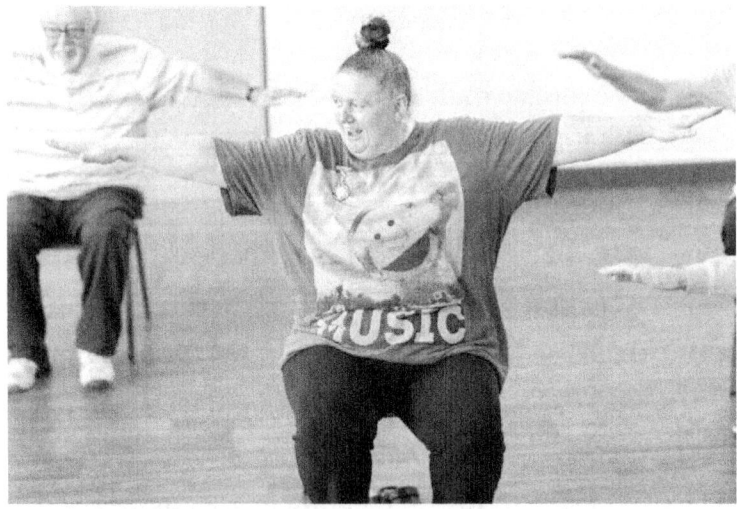

8. *Wrist rotation is a simple exercise that increases blood flow in your wrists. Source: https://www.pexels.com/photo/elderly-people-exercising-11674390/*

Standing without Help

Instructions:

1. Sit on a chair with no armrests and cross your arms.

2. While sitting, lean slightly forward and put your weight on your legs.

3. Stand up with your arms still crossed, then sit down.

4. Repeat 5 to 10 times.

Ankles Alphabets

This warm-up improves your ankle's mobility and increases its strength.

Instructions:

1. Sit in an upright position, placing your palms on your thighs with your feet on the floor.

2. Lift your right leg.

3. Pretend your big toe is a pen, and write the alphabet in the air.

4. Don't move your leg, only your foot.

5. Alternate with the other foot.

Seated Marches

This warm-up improves mobility and flexibility in the thighs and hips and elevates your heart rate.

Instructions:

1. Sit up straight on a chair and place both arms by your side with your feet on the floor hip-width apart.

2. Squeeze the muscles in your belly to engage core muscles.

3. Lift your left leg as high as you can but keep your knee bent.

4. Slowly lower your left foot to the floor.

5. Repeat the previous steps with your right foot.

Setting Up Your Stretching Space

You need to assign a tidy and spacious place for stretching. It should be an inviting and cozy space to motivate you to exercise every day.

Choose a Bright and Tidy Space

Stretching exercises can be challenging. There will be days when you would rather sit and watch TV than exercise. This happens to everyone, so you need to give yourself a push. Make sure your stretching space is clean and well-lit. It would be ideal if you could find a place near a window so you can get natural light. Put a decorative lamp in your stretching space or hang string lights if you don't have access to natural light. Light is significant to get you energized and ready for exercising. A poorly lit room will make you feel lazy and sleepy.

Some stretching exercises require you to lean against a wall or lie on the floor, so make sure to keep your exercise space tidy. If you have to clean or tidy up every time you want to exercise, you will keep putting it off and, in turn, give up on stretching altogether. Clean it every chance you get, or hire someone to do it for you. A clean space will keep you focused. Clutter and dust affect the mind and make you stressed, which isn't the best environment for exercising. Remove unnecessary objects and keep your space organized. This gives you more room to stretch and makes it easier to find your equipment.

Face the Room, Not the Wall

No one wants to look at a wall while exercising. This can be very boring, right? Set your exercising space to face the room or, even better, a window. If this isn't possible, consider stretching in front of a mirror. You will be able to see yourself and the room, which will be more interesting.

Avoid cracked mirrors as they will distort your reflection, giving you a headache and making it hard to focus. Don't stretch near cracked walls either because they can impact your energy.

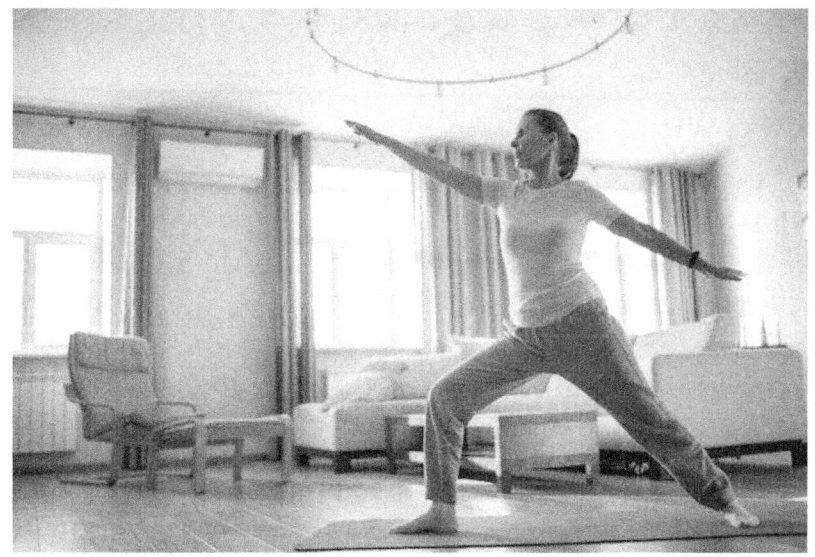

9. *Set your exercising space to face the room, or even better, a window. Source: https://www.pexels.com/photo/an-elderly-woman-doing-a-yoga-6975757/*

Close the Door

You must be focused while stretching, especially if there are moves you need to remember. So, close the door while exercising to eliminate distractions. You should also assign the space away from the door so you won't hear children playing or phones ringing. Make your space as quiet as possible.

You should always avoid walkways and hallways so you won't be constantly interrupted.

Stay Clear from Dropped Ceilings and Beams

Your stretching area should be spacious. Beams and dropped ceilings limit your movements, so it will make it difficult to stretch your body. Choose an open space with high ceilings so you can stretch easily and freely.

Test the space before choosing it by doing some stretching exercises to see if your legs and arms will touch or knock anything.

Add Plants

Stretching outdoors isn't accessible to everyone, so how about bringing the outdoors indoors? Decorate your stretching space with plants to liven it up and make it more inviting. Plants also increase the oxygen in the air, which is good for your physical and mental health, especially if you are doing deep breathing exercises while stretching.

Choose any plants. You can even opt for flowers to add color to the room. However, if you don't know much about plants or don't have time to care for them, you can get an aloe plant, a pretty plant with long leaves which requires little care and can transform the room. Other low-maintenance plants include succulents, Christmas cacti, and snake plants.

Create a Positive Space

Your stretching space should make you feel good while exercising. If you feel bored, sad, or frustrated, will you exercise again? Of course not. Remember, this is your space, so you can make it whatever you like. Look at the space and ask yourself, "How can I make it better?" What do you need to add or change to motivate you to exercise every day? Do you need to remove some objects and declutter? Is there something in the room elevating your stress or anxiety? Make the necessary changes and organize your space to make it aesthetically pleasing and inviting. You can create positive vibes in the room by hanging art, a motivational mantra, or a quote on the wall, or you can turn on music.

Dedicate a Space Solely to Stretching

Understandably, you can't assign a whole room for stretching. So, whichever space you choose, dedicate it only to exercising. It will make it easier for you to remain focused and mentally prepare you for stretching. When you associate a space with a single activity, it can become a habit. Every time you walk into the room, you will only think about stretching.

Necessary Stretching Equipment

Although stretching is considered low maintenance and doesn't require much equipment, there are a few things you need in your home for effective exercise.

Yoga Mat

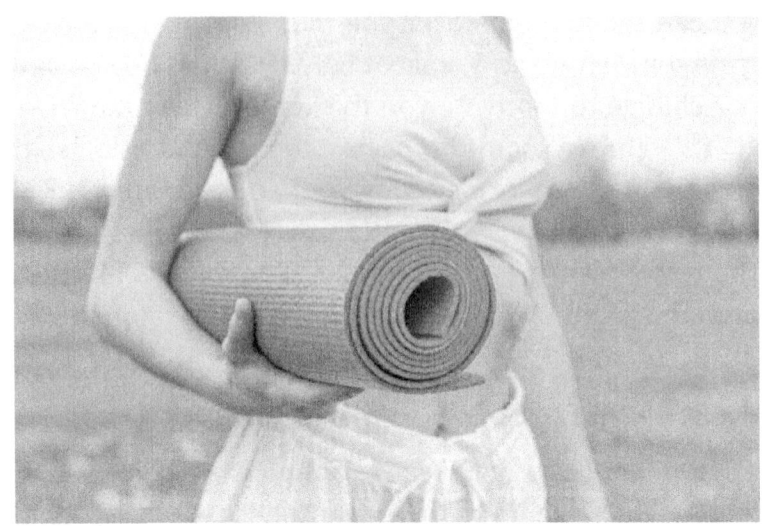

10. A yoga mat is the most significant piece of stretching equipment.
Source: https://www.pexels.com/photo/woman-standing-and-holding-blue-yoga-mat-2394051/

A yoga mat is the most significant piece of stretching equipment. Yoga mats are cheap, simple, easy to store, and make exercising easier and more effective. You can perform all forms of stretches on the mat. It enhances your balance and helps you strengthen your core. You can use it anywhere around the house, and it won't take up much space since you can store it anywhere.

Choose a yoga mat you love and can easily work with to motivate you to exercise. There are different types, shapes, widths, and colors to choose from, so take your time to look around until you find the right one. Your yoga mat should be comfortable and pretty to make stretching easy and fun.

If you want a mat that supports your knees, look for a thick one. Although it's easier to buy online, it's better to buy a mat from a store so you can feel the texture. Make sure it feels soft and comfortable. Remember to keep your mat clean.

Resistance Bands

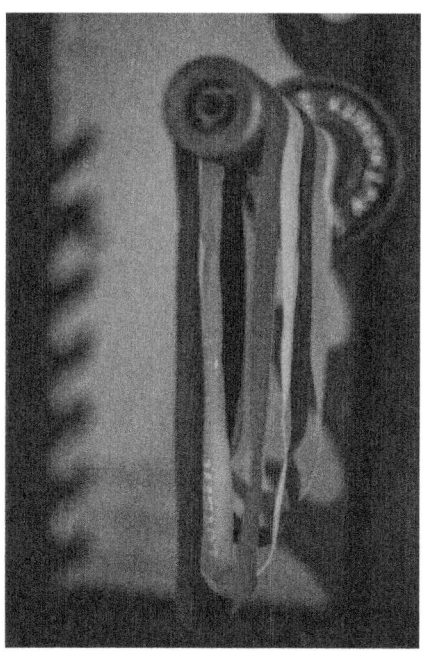

11. Resistance bands are necessary because they can be incorporated into many stretching techniques. Source: https://unsplash.com/photos/blue-green-and-yellow-coated-wires-Mzu7qcmP5tk

Resistance bands are versatile, cheap, and light tools. These bands are necessary because they can be incorporated into many stretching techniques. They apply tension to the muscles to increase your strength, boost coordination, enhance mobility, and reduce the risk of injury.

Choose a high-quality band. Thick bands are your best option because they are durable and don't snap or get sticky. They are made from rubber or elastic. There isn't a right or wrong choice. Merely choose the one you prefer.

Whether you are a beginner or experienced, you can work with resistance bands.

Chair

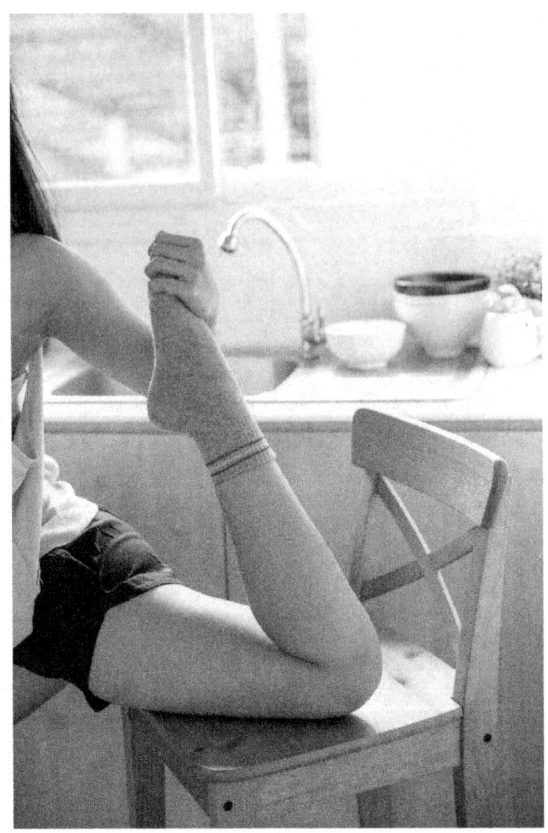

12. Stay clear from armchairs or chairs with wheels. Source: https://www.pexels.com/photo/person-s-leg-on-a-wooden-chair-7592321/

Put a stable chair with a straight back, like a kitchen chair, in your stretching area to hold onto for balance. Stay clear from armchairs or chairs with wheels. You might feel unsteady while stretching, especially if you are a beginner and working on your flexibility and muscle strength. Having something to hold on to will reduce the risk of injury.

Water Bottle

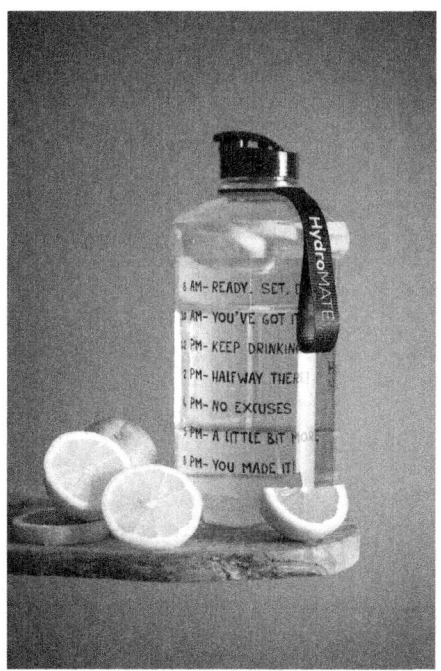

13. You must stay hydrated while exercising. Source: https://www.pexels.com/photo/slice-lemon-beside-glass-pitcher-on-wooden-table-3766180/

It is vital that you have a water bottle near you while stretching. You must stay hydrated while exercising.

It is essential that you don't start stretching without being prepared. Find a quiet place at home, solely for stretching, with no distractions. Buy the necessary equipment and place them in your stretching space. Learn a few warm-up exercises and perform them every time before you exercise to avoid injuries and prepare yourself mentally and physically before stretching.

Chapter 3: Upper Body Stretches

Your upper body is used for a lot, so keeping it flexible and mobile will greatly impact your independence as you age. Stretching is a core component of working out, and regular exercise helps maintain functionality. If you don't use it, you may lose it. Engaging all your muscles with deep stretches is an activating force that reintroduces you to your body. To get the enriching, positive benefits the combination of exercise and stretching provides, targeting specific groups so that you do not neglect any part of your body is advisable. Zooming into the upper body with focused stretches contributes to the complex puzzle of your physical health.

Neck and Shoulder Stretches

The constant sitting of a sedentary lifestyle can harshly impact your neck and shoulders. Nerve compression, injuries, and muscle strain contribute to pain and limited movement in your upper body. Using these upper body stretches in conjunction with an active life will help loosen you up to do the hands-on activities you desire. The pain relief and flexibility you gain by introducing upper body exercises into your stretching routine are unmatched.

Years of working could have had an impact on your neck and shoulders, but you can do remedial work to restore the area and increase your comfort exponentially. There are numerous causes for tension in your neck and shoulders, but they can be counteracted with a few targeted minutes of stretching daily. The following exercises are designed to gently stretch your neck and shoulders in ways that are safe and effective. The following easy exercises can be quickly grasped to introduce them into your routine immediately.

Neck Retraction

Since many people spend most of their time slouched over in a terrible posture, whether working at a desk, in a workshop, or watching TV, counteracting the damage caused by this position is essential. Just a few minutes of performing some neck retractions will help you correct your posture and release some tension as a result of repeated contortion of your neck. This stretch is gentle and relaxing, so it is perfect for a beginner or someone with mobility issues.

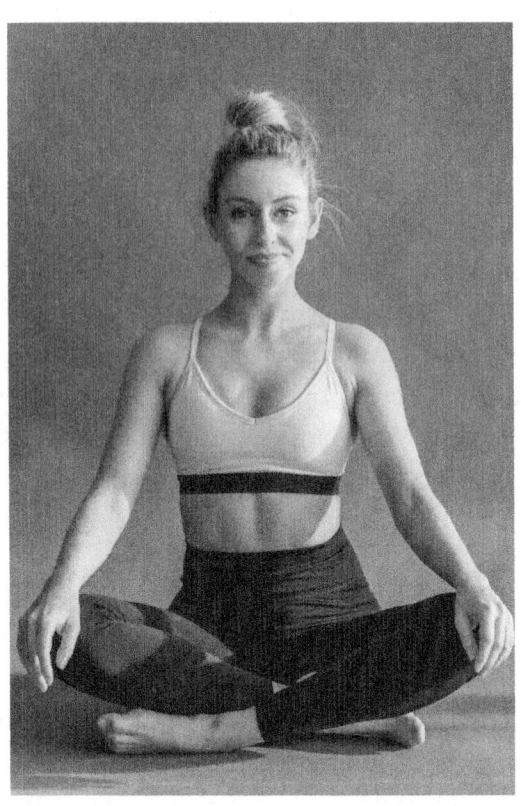

14. *This stretch is gentle and relaxing, so it is perfect for a beginner or someone with mobility issues. Source: https://www.pexels.com/photo/fit-woman-practicing-easy-sit-posture-6454159/*

- Start this stretch standing up or in a seated position, depending on what you are comfortable with.

- Keep your back straight as you look forward in a relaxed position. Make sure you are not stiff or clenching any muscles in your neck, shoulders, or face.

- Slowly move your head all the way forward as far as you can while keeping your back in the same position.

- Hold that stretch for about five seconds.

- Release the stretch gently as you move your head back.

- Now, tuck your chin into your chest as far as you can and lean slightly backwards without looking up or down instead, keep your eyes facing the front.

- Hold this stretch for five seconds.

- Repeat this stretch about three times for maximum effectiveness.

Neck Rotation

There are twenty muscles in your neck, all attached to a network of bones and tendons. Your neck supports your head, which is the control room of the body, so it has an important job to do. The complicated structure of the neck and its constant use can cause it to get injured or strained quite often. Neck rotations give each muscle attention and untangle the knotted mess resulting from overusing the neck and subjecting it to decades of ill-treatment. This simple stretch is an amazing way to start your stretch routine and gym sessions because it is calming and provides an instant sense of relief.

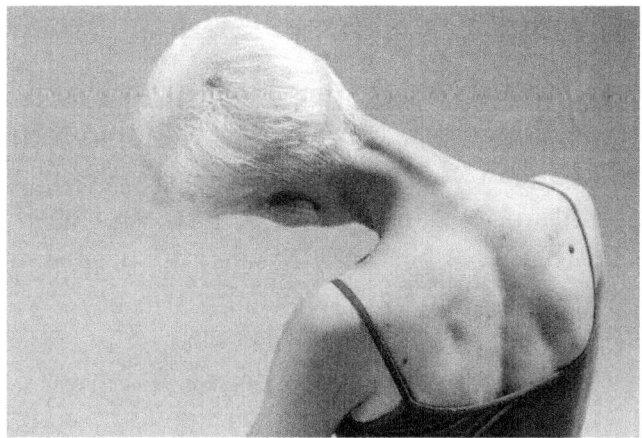

15. Neck rotations give each muscle attention and untangle the knotted mess resulting from overusing the neck and subjecting it to decades of ill-treatment. Source: https://www.pexels.com/photo/woman-in-black-spaghetti-strap-top-9486637/

- Start this stretch in a standing or sitting position. Switch between standing and sitting and see what feels best for you because listening to your body is an important part of stretching.

- Slowly lean your head down until you are looking at the ground, then rotate your head to the left.

- From the left position, continue rotation until your head is leaning back.

- Now, continue the motion toward the right and back down to the center.

- Repeat the same motion in the opposite direction.

- Make sure to be deliberate and slow with your movements so you reach each muscle in your neck.

- Do about three to five rotations on each side.

- Moving slowly and gently is important because you do not want to make abrupt movements and get injured.

Shoulder Rolls

Lifting something heavy, sleeping in an awkward position, or even typing can cause excruciating pain that feels like it's tucked away under your shoulder so deeply that you cannot reach it. Continuous damage to this area can cause so much discomfort that you become frozen and unable to move. Proper motion in your shoulders helps you move your arms and lift things in various positions. Therefore, maintaining shoulder health is paramount to the work you do with your hands. Shoulder rolls help prevent the build-up of inflammation in your muscles and stretch your tendons so that you can swing your arms freely.

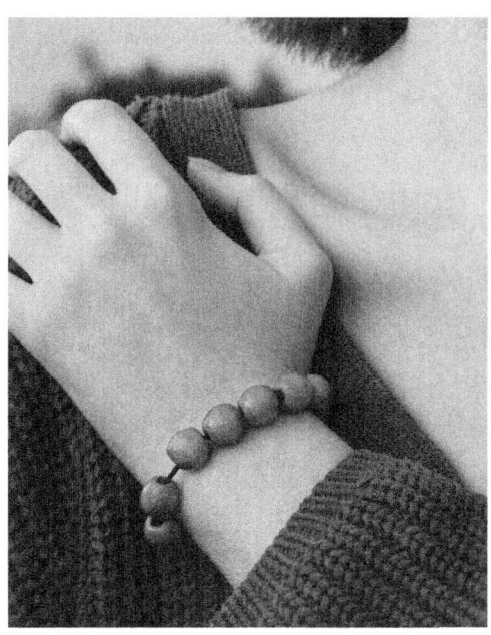

16. Shoulder rolls help prevent the build-up of inflammation in your muscles. Source: https://www.pexels.com/photo/wooden-bracelet-of-red-beads-19092856/

- Stand with your feet spread comfortably about the width of your hips.

- Make sure that your knees aren't locked and are slightly bent to prevent joint injuries.

- Let your arms hang loosely next to your body.

- Take a deep breath and lift your shoulders to the ceiling.

- Now that your shoulders are lifted sky high, rotate them back and squeeze your shoulder blades together.

- Exhale as you slowly bring your shoulders back to their natural resting position, then move them forward so that your upper back is humped, then release them back to neutral.

- Repeat this stretch about ten times.

- You can alternate the movement by rotating your shoulders backward and then forward.

- Over time, this exercise will increase your range of motion.

Pendulum Stretch

The pendulum stretch is a fun exercise focusing on your shoulders and stretching your entire back. This exercise is a gravity-assisted stretch that increases your mobility and range of motion while relieving pain and increasing recovery time after sustaining shoulder injuries. This stretch is great if you have hurt your rotator cuff or undergone shoulder surgery. The exercise is recommended by doctors because of its impact on the healing process.

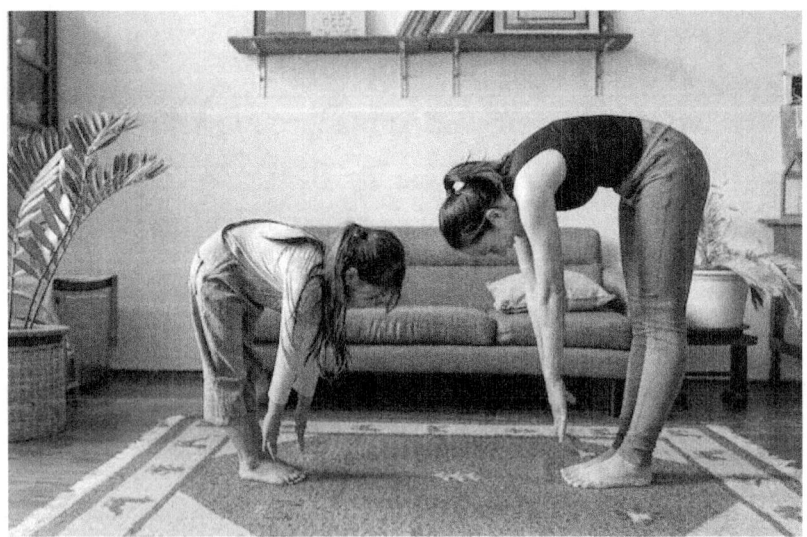

17. *This exercise is a gravity-assisted stretch that increases your mobility. Source: https://www.pexels.com/photo/photo-of-woman-and-girl-stretching-their-body-4473608/*

- For this exercise, you will need a chair, bench, or table for support.

- Stand with the bench on the right side of your body.

- Stand with your feet at about hip-width and lean forward until you are looking at the ground with your body at almost a 90-degree angle, resting your right arm on the bench.

- Swing your left arm back and forth, and rotate it in different directions, making circular motions with your hand.

- Gravity will help you stretch your shoulder.

- Move your arm around for about thirty seconds before switching sides and repeating the exercise.

- As gravity pulls your arm downward, you will feel your shoulder blade open up.

Cross-Body Shoulder Stretch

The cross-body shoulder stretch works on the posterior shoulder, which helps you increase how well you can move your arms. In addition to relieving pain, the stretch also decreases the risk of injury and can help you restore your posture that may have been distorted over the years. The exercise allows a deep stretch that engages many muscle groups and joints around your shoulders.

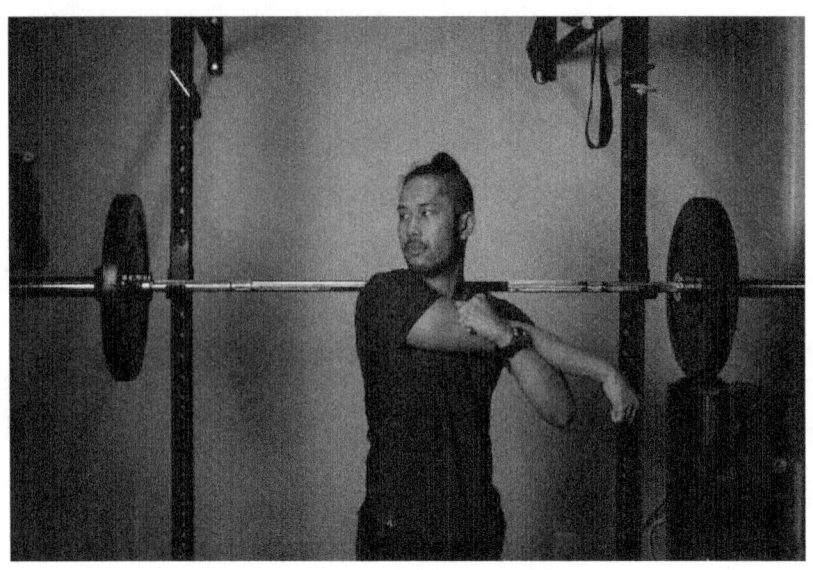

18. The stretch decreases the risk of injury. Source: https://www.pexels.com/photo/man-in-blue-crew-neck-t-shirt-stretching-12890895/

- Start in a standing position, making sure your body is relaxed, and your feet are about hip-width apart.

- When doing these standing stretches, ground your feet so that you are stable and balanced.

- Lift your right arm extending in front of you, palm facing the ground.

- Reach your arm across your chest so that your right hand is on the left side of your body.

- Now bend your left arm, placing your forearm across your right arm.

- With your left fist pointed at the ceiling, use your forearm to pull your right arm toward your chest, keeping your right arm straight.

- Hold the stretch for about twenty seconds.

- Release and switch sides to repeat the stretch.

Arm and Wrist Stretches

Your arms and hands are probably the body parts you consciously use the most often. From grabbing your glasses on the table to read and making yourself a cup of tea, it seems that your hands and arms are busy all day. The constant use of your arms and hands makes it more likely that you will develop muscles and joint pain or sustain an injury. By keeping your arms limber, you ensure that they are always ready for use. As people age, pain and stiffness cause them to drop things a lot more and be generally clumsier. Stretching your arms and wrists enables you to perform strength and precision movements for years. Stretching is like the oil of the muscles and joints, so tunnel into those painful crevasses of your arms to get the relief you deserve and build the mobility to elevate your wellness.

Wrist Stretch

The precise motions you make, like holding a spoon, writing, or using your phone, impact your wrist. Nerve and joint pain are common in wrists because of the repetitive movements the body part goes through regularly. Wrist pain can be limiting because it stops you from participating in numerous activities. Therefore, a basic wrist stretch can help you reduce the excruciating pain holding you back from living your life on your terms.

Although you can complete this exercise while seated, for best results, the wrist stretch should be done standing.

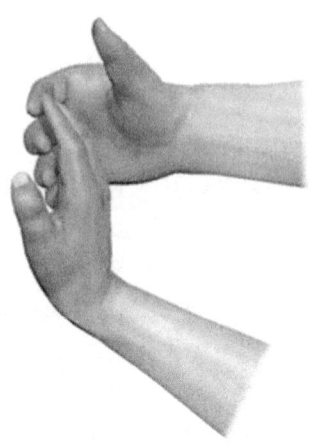

Wrist Flexor Stretch

19. *Nerve and joint pain are common in wrists because of the repetitive movements the body part goes through regularly. Source: BruceBlaus, CC BY-SA 4.0 <https://creativecommons.org/licenses/by-sa/4.0>, via Wikimedia Commons: https://commons.wikimedia.org/wiki/File:Exercise_Wrist_Flexor _Stretch.png*

- Stand straight up with your legs spread in a comfortable stance.

- Extend one arm in front of you with your palm facing up.

- Grab your fingers with the opposite hand and gently bend your fingers down toward the ground.

- You should repeat this three times for each hand, holding the stretch for five seconds before releasing it and switching hands.

- Another variation is facing your palm downward and then repeating the same exercise.

Clenched Fist Stretch

Your hands are filled with bones and tendons arranged in a beautiful matrix of interlocking parts. Stretching should consider how each tiny section of your hand interacts to perform daily tasks. Think of the infinite combination of wrist and finger movements you use regularly, from picking up a penny from the ground to opening a drawer or playing an instrument. These grips target various muscles in your hand and use different tendons. The clenched fist exercise is perfect for combining hand movements to stretch your forearm muscles and work on the tiny weaving parts inside your hand structure.

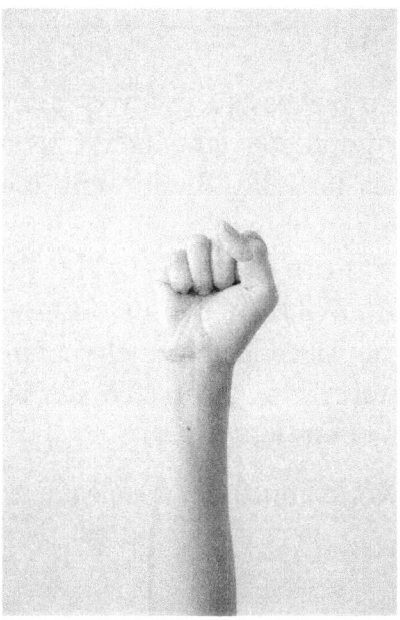

20. Stretching should consider how each tiny section of your hand interacts to perform daily tasks. Source: https://www.pexels.com/photo/close-up-of-a-clenched-fist-901757 9/

- Sit up in a chair with your feet on the ground and spread slightly apart.

- Gently rest your open hands on your thighs with your palms turned to the sky.

- Curl your fingers until your hands are completely closed.

- With your forearms and elbows glued to your thighs, curl your clenched fists up and hold the stretch for five seconds.

- Do about 5 to 10 reps of this exercise.

- When you release and rest, you'll feel as if your forearms and wrists can breathe again as your blood flow increases.

Wall Bicep Stretch

Tension in your biceps can grab your attention throughout the day because simple movements like scratching your nose can become a hassle. Fully functioning biceps make going through the daily motions much easier. Moreover, with healthy biceps, you can do many hobbies that require your arms. Furthermore, you can lift anything without too much effort or pain. The wall bicep stretch is simple yet effective. With minimal strain, you can stretch all the sections of your bicep with an easy motion.

This stretch works multiple muscles, including your chest and shoulders.

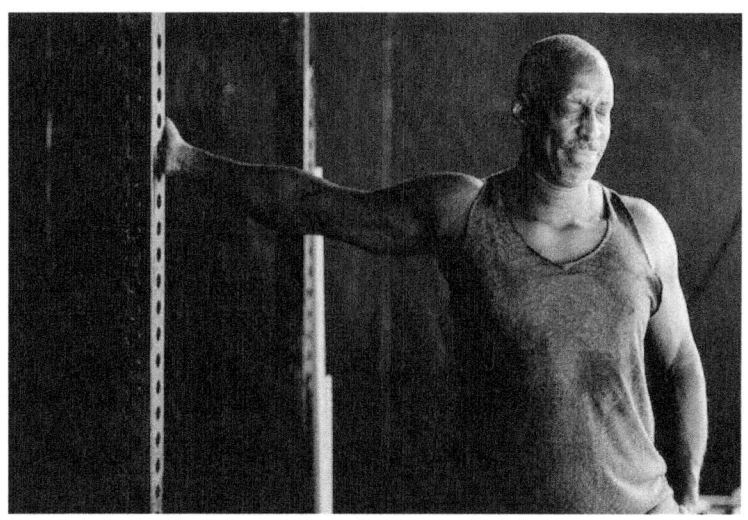

21. Fully functioning biceps make going through the daily motions much easier. Source: https://www.pexels.com/photo/photo-of-man-stretching-his-arm-4720286/

- Standing at a 90-degree angle perpendicular to the wall, lift your right arm at your side so that your hand lines up with your shoulder.

- With your arm extended fully, place your open palm on the wall and turn to your right, twisting your body until you feel the stretch in your bicep and chest.

- Hold this stretch for 15 to 30 seconds, then gently turn back to release.

- Switch hands and repeat the stretch for the other side.

- This stretch can be done anywhere, so you can use it whenever you feel discomfort in your chest, shoulders, or arms.

Triceps Stretch

The combination of the bicep and triceps is responsible for many of the arm's big movements. When your triceps are not stretched, it can cause spasms and tightness. The terrible pain can shoot from your elbow to your shoulder. Releasing some tension in your shoulders helps you lift better and will make your arm workouts more impactful.

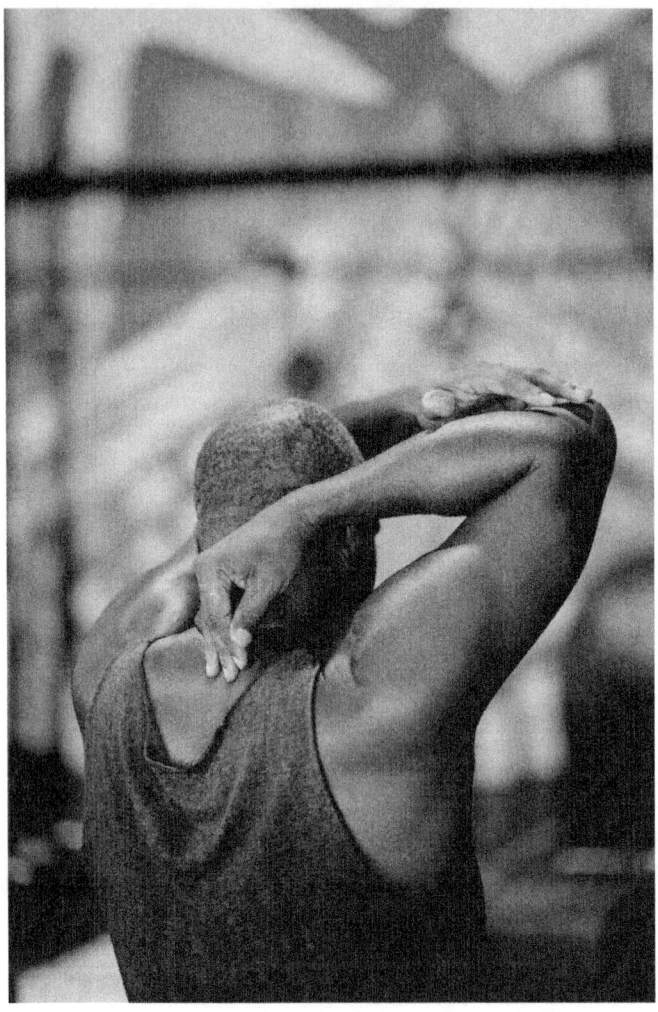

22. When your triceps are not stretched, it can cause spasms and tightness. Source: https://www.pexels.com/photo/shallow-focus-photo-of-man-stretching-4720259/

- Begin by standing straight up with your legs spread comfortably.

- Raise your arm straight up next to your ear.

- Bend your elbow to reach your hand to the center of your back.

- Use the opposite hand to press down on your elbow until you feel the stretch at the back of your arm.

- Hold this stretch for 15 to 20 seconds, then switch arms and repeat the process.

Chest and Upper Back Stretches

A tender chest can ruin your day. The muscles that form the chest are relatively large, so when you have pain, it cannot go unnoticed. Lifting yourself off the ground requires your chest muscles, so having the area limber will improve your well-being significantly. Your chest and your back are an overlapping weave of muscles aiding in sitting, standing, and a wide array of dynamic movements. A stiff back can be so debilitating that it causes you to lose sleep and make many of your daily activities miserable. Stretching the chest and upper back remedies a large family of muscles by getting the blood circulating and squeezing out lactic acid. Working on your chest and back will significantly improve your overall health because of the large area it covers and the constant work that involves these parts of your body.

Chest Opener

This standing stretch is one of the most helpful exercises you can do to address chest pain. This stretch opens up the heart and lung areas to get oxygen spreading through the body better, improving the cells' metabolism.

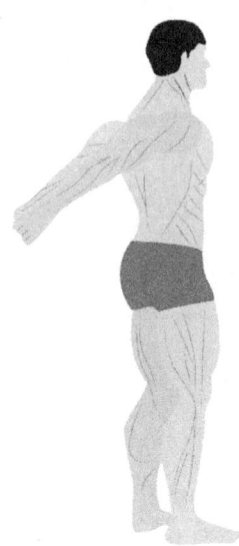

23. This stretch opens up the heart and lung areas to get oxygen spreading through the body better, improving the cells' metabolism. Source: https://cdn-cccio.nitrocdn.com/sQAAylIpwgMYZgBLSXcMgCkUIbfIzHvb/asset s/images/optimized/rev-b05b9eb/www.aleanlife.com/wp-content/uploads/2020/11/chest-stretch-arms-behind-back.jpg

- Begin in a standing position with your feet spread comfortably, hip-width.

- Reach behind your lower back and interlock your fingers.

- Pull your clasped hands up toward the ceiling.

- As you pull up your hands, tilt your head back as far as possible and look at the sky.

- Press your shoulder blades together as you get a deep stretch through your chest.

- This stretch can be felt in your shoulders and your spine.

- As you release the stretch, you will feel the oxygenated blood moving freely through your back and chest.

Neck and Chest Stretch

This is another stretch that combats the hunched-over lifestyle many people have. People stare at screens, eat crouched over a table, or look down when reading, impacting the muscles and joints as they become stiff in this terrible posture. Humans were designed to be in motion on the open savannas or climbing in the forest, so the constant sitting is against the natural functioning of the body. Hence, it must be addressed with consistent work. The neck and chest stretch works the muscles most affected by constant crouching.

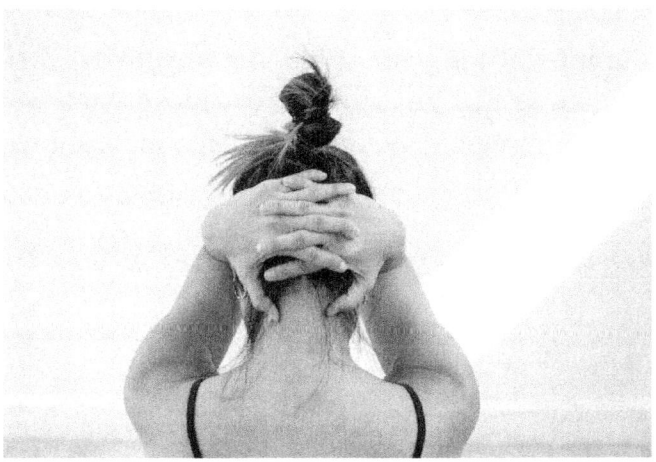

24. Humans were designed to be in motion on the open savannas or climbing in the forest, so the constant sitting is against the natural functioning of the body. Source: https://www.pexels.com/photo/unrecognizable-woman-stretching-neck-7593063/

- Start by sitting on a chair with your back erect. Spread your feet hip-width apart and place them firmly on the floor.

- Lift your hands behind your head as if you were being arrested.

- Slightly tilt your head back into your hands with your chin up.

- Take a deep breath in and lean to the right so that your elbow faces the ground.

- Hold this stretch for three seconds and inhale as you come back to the center.

- Repeat the cycle for the other side.

- You can do three to five repetitions of this exercise.

Seated Gentle Back Bend

Losing mobility in your spine is a tragedy because it can massively impact your ability to move independently. Therefore, embracing a routine that incorporates back stretching is advisable.

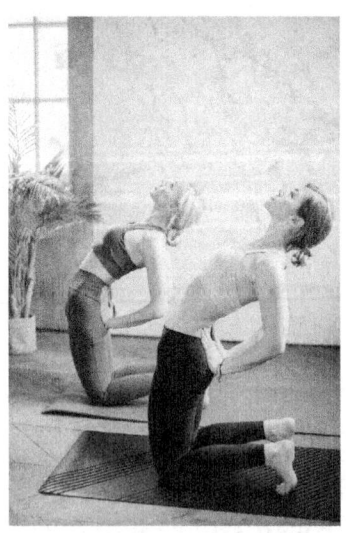

25. Losing mobility in your spine is a tragedy because it can massively impact your ability to move independently. Source: https://www.pexels.com/photo/women-practicing-yoga-3823151/

- To do a seated gentle back bend, sit upright on a chair.

- With your feet spread at hips width and placed firmly on the ground, put your hands on your lower back and lean your head up toward the sky.

- You should feel this stretch in your neck, shoulder blades, and mid-back.

- Since many people often slouch, this exercise directly counteracts that position and opens your chest up while flexing your spine.

Seated Cat and Cow

The seated cat and cow stretch is a variation of a popular yoga pose, adapted to be a little bit easier for beginners and people with mobility issues. This ancient movement is fluid and flowing, so it really gets the blood moving. The constant movement involved in the stretch uses multiple muscle groups at different moments, which helps your body coordinate so that you can make more dynamic movements.

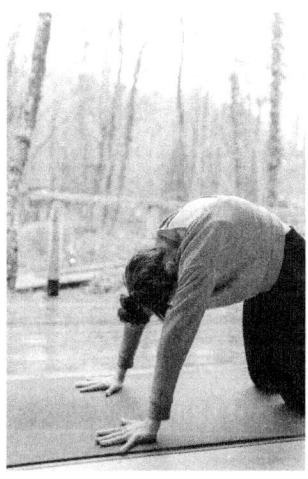

26. *This ancient movement is fluid and flowing, so it really gets the blood moving. Source: https://www.pexels.com/photo/a-person-doing-the-marjariasana-7663035/*

- Start by sitting upright, making sure your feet are spread as wide as your shoulders on the ground and facing forward.

- Lean forward slightly from your waist, placing your hands on your knees with your fingers facing the middle line of your body.

- Inhale as you arch your back, pushing your chest out toward the ceiling as high as you can.

- Exhale and round your back as you tuck your chin into your chest.

- Cycle through this movement about five times as you get an easy rhythm going.

- Do the motion slowly and deliberately so you can feel each section of your spine and your back and chest muscles with each repetition.

From simple tasks like eating to heavier lifting and even getting up from a seated or lying position, your upper body deeply impacts your everyday activities. The combination of a strength training routine and stretching exercises targeting all the various muscle groups from your waist to your neck allows you to maintain your functionality for years. The beauty of many upper body stretches is that you can do them anywhere. Stretching not only helps reduce pain in the upper body, but it also increases circulation and flexibility. Regularly stretching your arms, legs, core, shoulders, and back will help prevent injuries in these problematic areas. As you age, it is crucial to put in the additional work to maintain your body. After a quick morning warm-up, spend about fifteen minutes targeting your upper body with simple, specialized stretches to provide the daily rejuvenation you need to stay active and independent. The tension that leaves your body with stretching and conscious breathing is the mini-vacation you need to relax and relieve stress. Wellness practices often emphasize diet, cardio, and strength training, but without upper body stretching, you can derail your efforts because of injuries and reduced mobility.

Chapter 4: Lower Body Stretches

As you age, your body deteriorates, so you have to take additional steps for maintenance. One of your bodily functions that is affected when you are older is balance. Senior citizens are at a higher risk of falling than the average person. Stretching your lower body helps improve balance, increase stability, and participate in the activities that bring you joy. Keeping a solid center of gravity for stability will be improved by the increased strength and flexibility a regular stretching routine promotes.

Since your legs are the primary vehicle for getting around, stretching them well is essential to facilitate your independent movement. Arthritis is one of the most common ailments related to aging, impacting your knees, ankles, and many other joints. The following stretching exercises can help reduce the inflammation arthritis induces. Your range of motion will increase so you can use your body to its fullest potential. Your quality of life is significantly influenced by how well you move around, so stretching the legs that carry you will positively shift your well-being mentally and physically.

Leg Stretches

Following the correct safety protocols are crucial to continuously training and building a healthy stretching schedule. Hurting your legs will force you to be immobile or even bedridden, so make sure to warm up before you stretch. These leg stretches target the quads, calves, and hamstrings. Each section of your leg is equally important for sustaining fluid motion. Therefore, you should do a variety of stretches targeting each essential part. These muscle groups are activated when you walk. Therefore, the pain relief, mobility, and flexibility that are bolstered by daily practicing these stretches help keep you moving forward. Regularly engaging in these exercises will keep you on your feet for longer without needing to rest and lessen the risk of injury to counteract some of the negative effects of aging. Giving your legs some tender love and care with gentle stretching is part of the formula to live a healthy and active lifestyle.

Standing Quad Stretch

Depending on how good your balance is, you may need support like a table, chair, or wall to complete this stretch. If you are able to, you can do it without a chair, but be careful because you do not want to lose your balance and hurt yourself.

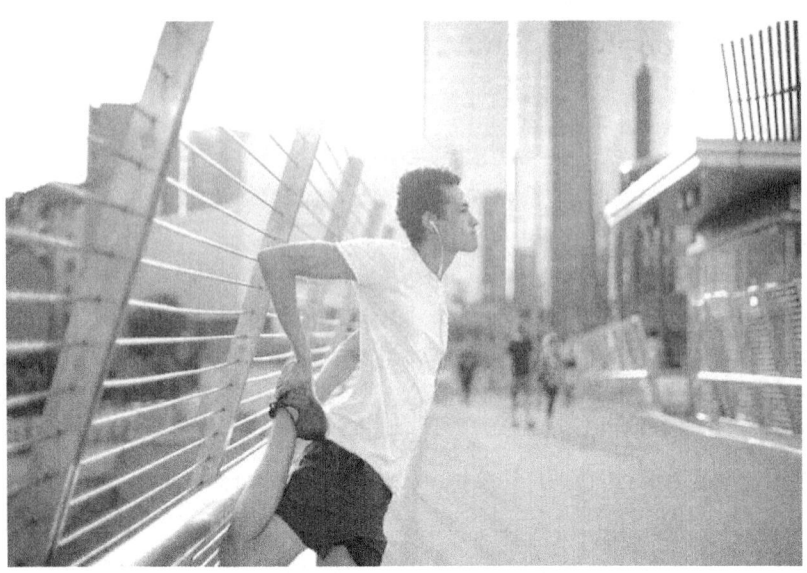

27. Be careful because you do not want to lose your balance and hurt yourself. Source: https://www.pexels.com/photo/focused-millennial-ethnic-athlete-in-earphones-listening-to-music-and-stretching-body-before-running-on-street-3799375/

- While standing up straight with your feet spread the width of your hips and holding onto your chair at the side of your body, slowly bend your right leg so that your heel touches your backside.

- Grab your right foot with your right hand and pull up and away from your body as far as possible.

- You should feel the tension of the stretch in your quad.

- Hold the tension for about 15 to 30 seconds and release, gently placing your foot down.

- It is important that your movements are slow and you do not allow gravity to drop your foot back into position, as sudden movements could cause injury.

- Switch legs and repeat the exercise.

Calf Stretch

Your calves support you when you are standing. They also have a big role in allowing you to position your feet differently while still maintaining balance. Stiff calves hugely influence the standing activities in which you can participate. Therefore, a good calf stretch can free you up to do so much more.

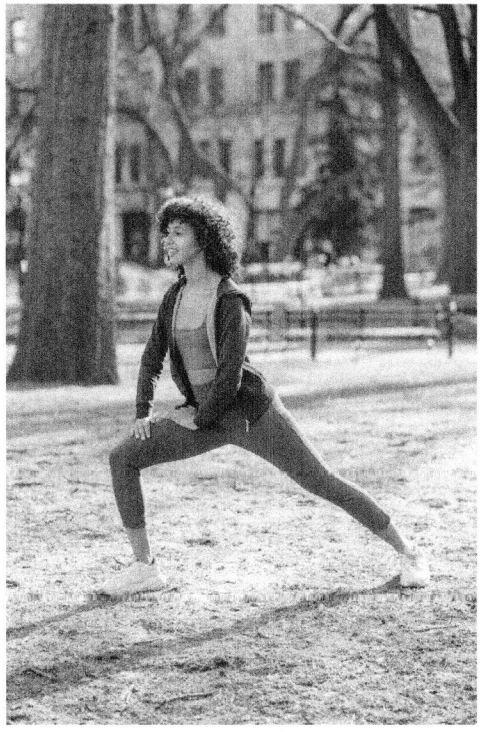

28. Stiff calves hugely influence the standing activities in which you can participate. Source: https://www.pexels.com/photo/fit-black-woman-stretching-legs-in-park-in-daylight-7242895/

- Position a chair, bench, table, or any comfortable support at about waist level at the side of your body.

- You can use a wall to support your balance if that feels better.

- Step your right foot forward about two feet, slightly bending your knees, and step back with your left foot, straightening your leg at a diagonal with your left heel staying flat on the floor.

- The further you bend your right knee and lean forward, the deeper the stretch into your left calf will be.

- Hold the stretch for about ten to twenty seconds, then switch legs to repeat.

- Listen to your body, and do not push yourself beyond your limits. Stretching causes discomfort, but it should not be excessively painful.

Standing Hamstring Stretch

For this exercise, you need a chair to hold onto. You should reserve this stretch for when you have a partner, or you can do it with your back to the wall for extra support if your balance is bad. The standing hamstring stretch pulls the back of your thigh to release tension in this region.

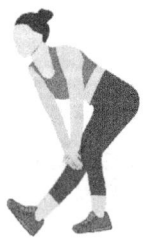

29. The standing hamstring stretch pulls the back of your thigh to release tension in this region. Source: https://publish.purewow.net/wp-content/uploads/sites/2/2020/05/best-hamstring-stretches-standing-hamstring-stretch.jpg?fit=728%2C524

- Stand upright with your feet firmly positioned about as wide as your hips.

- Place the chair to one side of you and hold onto it for balance.

- Step one leg slightly forward, keeping both heels on the ground.

- Relax your knee on the back leg, bending it slightly.

- Lean forward as you straighten your front leg, so it is diagonal, almost forming a triangle from the ground.

- You will feel the deep stretch at the back of your thigh.

- Hold the stretch for 10 to 20 seconds before relaxing back into an upright position.

- Switch legs and repeat.

Prone Quadricep Stretch

This stretch is great if you have low mobility or impaired balance because you are not standing but lying on the floor. Place a comfortable towel or exercise mat on the floor to begin. The area should be firm, not cushioned like a bed or couch.

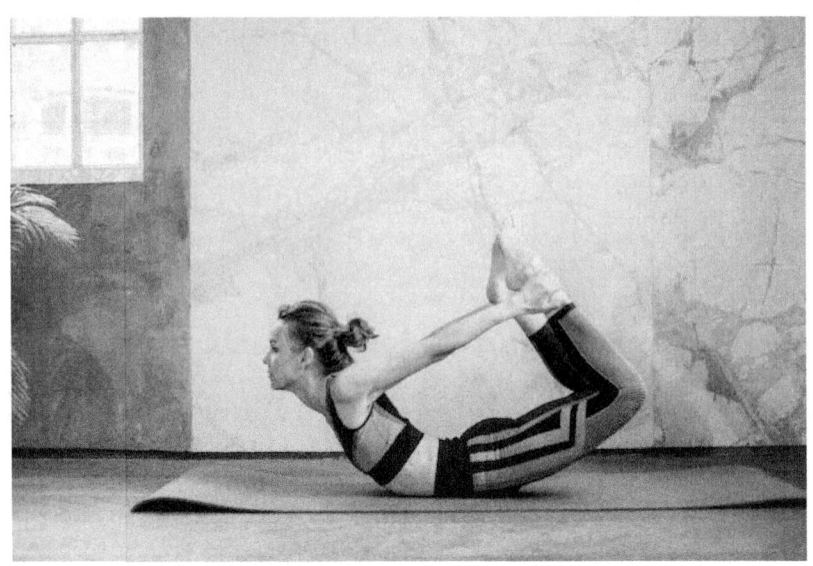

30. This stretch is great if you have low mobility or impaired balance because you are not standing but lying on the floor. Source: https://www.pexels.com/photo/woman-bow-pose-3822366/

- Begin the exercise by lying flat on your stomach with your body extended on the mat.

- Support yourself on your elbows, lift your head with the rest of your torso still touching the ground, and bend your right knee, reaching your heel toward the back of your neck as far as possible.

- Use your right hand to grab hold of your ankle and pull your leg toward your head while balancing on your left elbow.

- You might not be able to reach your ankle, which is okay.

- If you cannot grab your ankle, reach your arm back and lift your heel toward your head as far as possible.

- Hold the stretch for twenty seconds before switching sides.

- Remember, be careful when you get onto the floor and when getting up to prevent unnecessary injury.

Seated Hamstring Stretch

This variation of the hamstring stretch is perfect for people who are not comfortable standing and have low mobility.

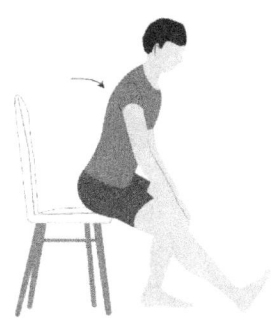

31. This variation of the hamstring stretch is perfect for people who are not comfortable standing and have low mobility. Source: https://i.pinimg.com/originals/2d/09/aa/2d09aa53e44eccc6fb68d f536cf7d8a1.png

- Begin this exercise by sitting upright on the edge of a chair with your feet spread the width of your hips.

- Place both your hands on your left knee as you extend your right leg in front of you and point your toes to the ceiling.

- One leg should be extended while the other leg, with your hands rested on it, should be bent.

- Lean forward from your waist, and you'll begin feeling your hamstring elongate.

- Keep your back straight when you lean forward.

- The further you lean, the deeper the stretch will be.

- Hold the position for about 20 seconds before relaxing and switching sides.

- This stretch can be done in the morning as a routine to get out of bed.

- The gentle stretch is easy to do and does not require much balance or motion to complete.

Hip and Glute Stretches

Much like your legs, or even more so, your hips and glutes (gluteal muscles, the group of muscles that make up the buttock area) are responsible for how well you balance. So, doing exercises to strengthen them and keep them limber will enable you to significantly reduce your risk of falling. Furthermore, the inflexibility of your hips causes lower back pain. Your glutes are the biggest muscles in your body, which is surprising considering they are often overlooked. Keeping your glutes flexible and the circulation moving through the large muscle assists with your overall comfort. The influence of balance, motion, and strength of the hips and glutes have made the muscle grouping central to the everyday functioning of the body. The glutes are formed from three muscles, namely, the gluteus maximus, gluteus medius, and gluteus minimus, so your stretch routine must target them all. The hip muscles comprise four groups defined according to how they relate to the hip joints. The four regions of hip muscles are the adductor, gluteal, iliopsoas, and lateral rotator groups. The following exercises target all the sections of your glutes and hip muscles.

Standing Hip Flexor

This exercise is immeasurably helpful for older people who have problems with lower back pain. By performing a standing hip flexor, you stabilize your core, which is great for balance and pulling and pushing movements. You can use a wall or a chair as balancing assistance with this stretch.

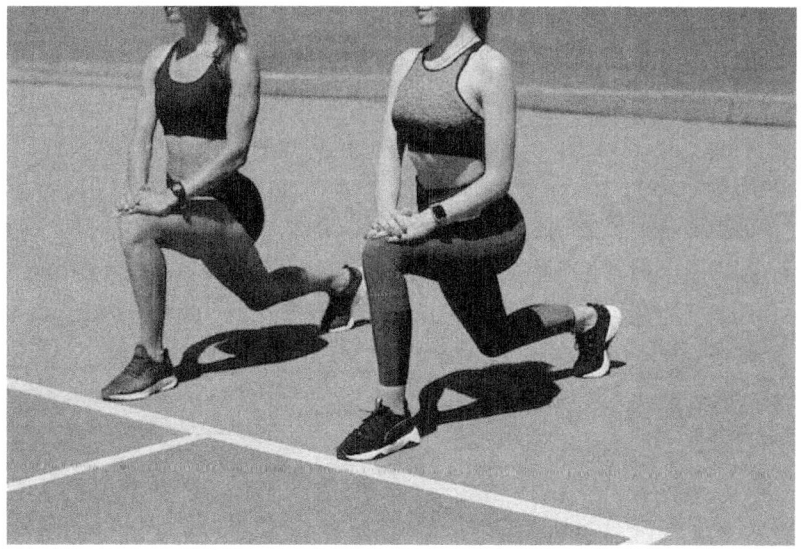

32. This exercise is immeasurably helpful for older people who have problems with lower back pain. Source: https://www.pexels.com/photo/two-women-doing-stretching-4348626/

- Stand up straight with your feet hip-width apart, placing your hands on your hips.

- Step one foot about an arm's length forward.

- Slowly bend your back leg as you descend to the ground until your knee touches the floor and your back heel is lifted.

- Your front foot should be firmly planted flat on the ground.

- Lean slightly forward and squeeze your glutes, holding the position for about thirty seconds.

- You can push the hold up to a minute if you feel able to.

- Slowly rise to a standing position to reset, and then repeat the exercise with your other leg as the front foot.

Butterfly Pose

This gentle and easy stretch should not be underestimated, and you will feel the tension deep inside your hips. Many yoga instructors have used the butterfly pose as a calm way for people to open their hip area and pelvis muscles for a tension-relieving stretch. This powerful pose works on both your flexors and abductors, so it helps loosen up your groin area, providing relief to your lower back and improving the flexibility in your inner thighs.

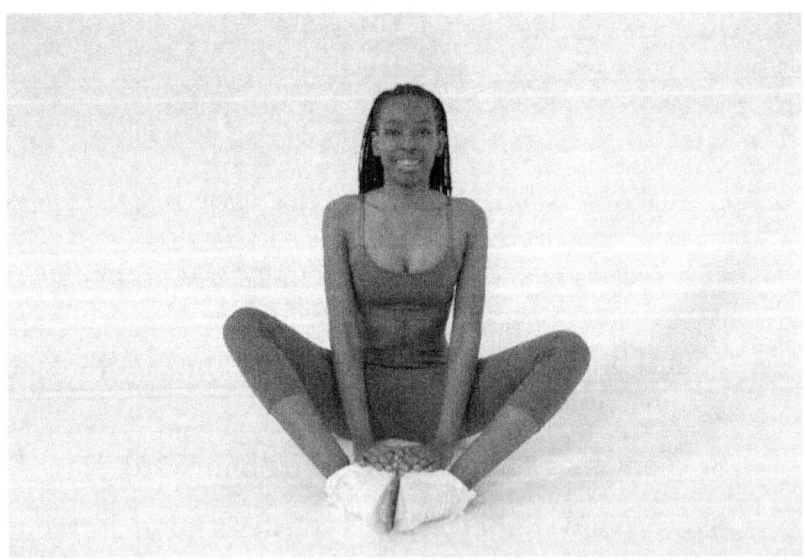

33. *Many yoga instructors have used the butterfly pose as a calm way for people to open their hip area and pelvis muscles for a tension-relieving stretch. Source: https://www.pexels.com/photo/fit-black-woman-sitting-in-baddha-konasana-pose-6311694/*

- Start by sitting flat on the ground with your gaze set forward, keeping your back straight and your head lifted high.

- Sit as if you are going to cross your legs, but instead, place the bottoms of your feet together and align to the center of your body.

- While keeping your back straight, grab your feet with both hands and lean forward.

- The combination of gravity pulling your knees down and the tension created by your lean feels like a breath of fresh air as the circulation in your lower body is increased.

- Hold the pose for about a minute before gently standing up to relax and shake out the tension.

Knee-to-Shoulder Stretch

The knee-to-shoulder stretch can be performed in the morning after a little warm-up when you get out of bed. This stretch targets your hips and thighs to give you more mobility. Furthermore, the stretch is done lying down, so there is less of a risk of injury or falling. Unless you have chronic pain or severe mobility issues, this relatively easy exercise can be done unassisted most of the time.

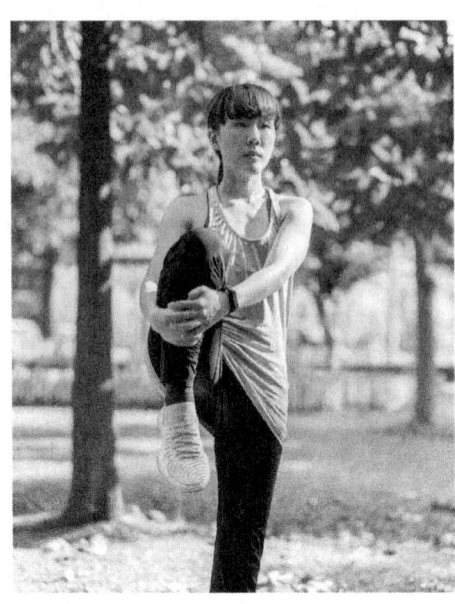

34. This stretch targets your hips and thighs to give you more mobility. Source: https://www.pexels.com/photo/determined-sportswoman-stretching-legs-in-summer-park-4426459/

- Start by lying flat on the floor on your back. It helps to have an exercise mat or something soft on the floor for comfort.

- Bend your knee as you raise your right leg to your chest while lying on the floor.

- Wrap your hand around your shin just below your knee and pull your leg toward your chest.

- Hold this position for twenty seconds before releasing and repeating the motion with your other leg.

- Once you are done with the stretch, keep lying down for a few seconds and feel how the stretch impacted your body as you take a few deep breaths.

Seated Figure-Four Stretch

This stretch can be a little difficult if you experience diminished mobility, but it is a seated exercise, so you do not have to worry too much about losing your balance. Another name for this exercise is the pigeon pose. It is a seated figure-four stretch that penetrates deep into the thigh muscles and glutes while loosening your hips. The variety of muscles and joints that the stretch strengthens is the perfect formula for lower body maintenance and rejuvenation.

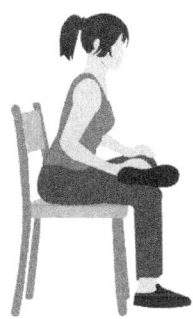

35. *It is a seated figure-four stretch that penetrates deep into the thigh muscles and glutes while loosening your hips. Source: https://www.wikihow.com/images/thumb/8/88/Do-a-Seated-Figure-Four-Step-6-Version-2.jpg/v4-460px-Do-a-Seated-Figure-Four-Step-6-Version-2.jpg*

- Sit with your back in an erect position on a comfortable, solid chair. Your feet should be facing forward while being spread about as wide as your hips

- Lift your right leg and place your ankle across your left knee.

- Grab onto your right shin with both hands and lean forward while maintaining the straightness in your back.

- Keep the stretch for thirty seconds before returning to your resting position.

- Repeat the exercise on your other leg.

- Be careful not to lean too far forward so that you fall off the chair or injure your muscles.

Cobra Stretch

The cobra stretch is a yoga pose that has been used for millennia. The stretch is almost miraculous with its bountiful benefits. Not only does the cobra pose reduce stress and improve posture, but it also helps with circulation and loosens your back, shoulders, and hips.

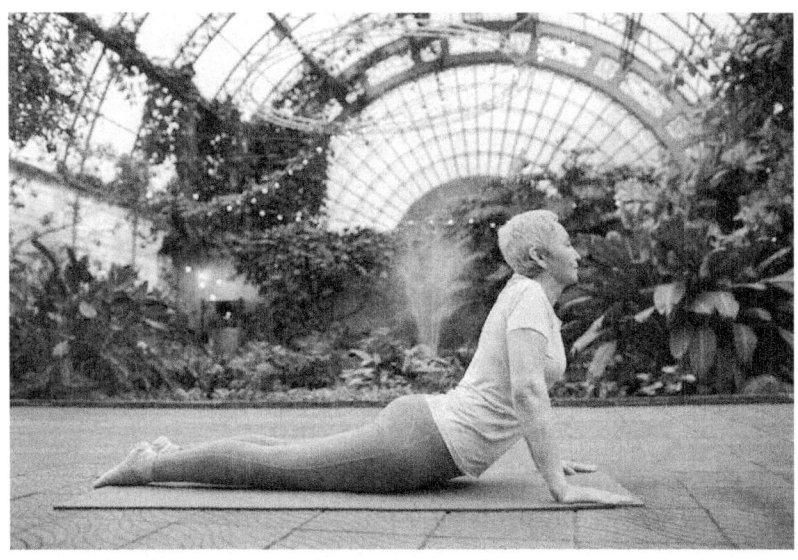

36. The stretch is almost miraculous with its bountiful benefits. Source: https://www.pexels.com/photo/woman-doing-cobra-pose-6787216/

- Begin by lying on the ground flat on your stomach.

- If your hips are stiff, you can place a pillow under your pelvis for support.

- Slowly raise your head, then your chest, and lastly, your stomach off the ground as you support your body with your arms. Your arms should be positioned next to your body in line with your shoulders.

- You are mimicking a cobra that is preparing to strike.

- Repeat this motion three times. Hold the stretch for approximately thirty seconds, then slowly return to a laying posture.

- Remember to inhale as you rise and exhale as you release so that your lungs can get involved to open your airways to get increased oxygen into your blood.

Ankle and Foot Stretches

Your ankle and feet are a complicated weave of bones, muscles, and tendons that help you move and balance. As you age, a lot of the flexibility in your ankles and feet is lost. This loss of flexibility significantly impacts your balance. Your ankle mobility is directly correlated to your risk of falling because stiff ankles and feet are a huge detriment to stability. Therefore, stretching and exercising your ankles and feet is essential to maintaining the balance to remain independent. Doing regular stretches every day will improve your quality of life because you will move and stand better. The stretches for your ankles and feet have a huge impact but are not difficult. Just a few minutes a day of ankle and foot stretches can make a big difference to your mobility. To counteract the loss of flexibility, you must do stretches and exercises that help all the intricate connections of your feet and ankles to work well together.

Toe Raise, Point, and Curl

Your toes seem so insignificant, but if you walk barefoot, you can see all the work they do. Just for an experiment, take off your shoes and move around a little to see how your toes assist in your motion and balance. Keeping your toes in shape is central to moving freely. The toe raise, point, and curl exercise includes a combination of movements.

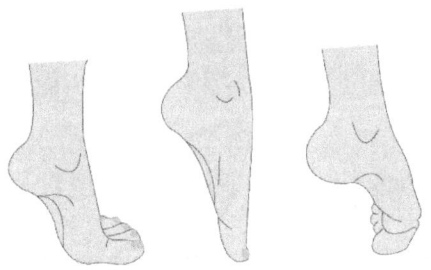

37. Keeping your toes in shape is central to moving freely. Source: https://s3assets.skimble.com/assets/1438475/image_iphone.jpg

- Start by sitting in a comfortable seat with your feet flat on the floor and hip-width apart.

- Raise your heels until only the balls of your feet are on the ground.

- Keep this position for about ten seconds.

- Next, raise your heels again, but this time, instead of the balls of your feet making contact with the ground, it should be the tips of your two big toes.

- Now, raise your heels as you curl your toes so that the tops of your toes are tucked underneath your feet.

- Lastly, keep your heels on the floor as you point your toes to the ceiling.

- Hold each position for five seconds.

Toe Extension

This stretch requires you to get a bit hands-on.

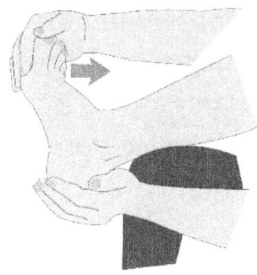

38. Get creative with this stretch and find what feels good. Source: https://api.kramesstaywell.com/Content/6066ca30-310a-4170-b001-a4ab013d61fd/ucr-images-v1/Images/hands-holding-foot-doing-toe-extension-exercise-358991

- Sit up straight in a comfortable chair with your feet spread hip-width flat on the ground.

- Lift your right foot, resting your ankle on your thigh.

- Grab your toes with your right hand and pull them back as far as they can go.

- You should feel the stretch in your toes and the bottom of your foot.

- Hold the stretch for twenty seconds before relaxing and repeating the exercise on your other foot.

- There are many tiny bones in your feet that flex and move according to how you walk, stand, or run.

- To get deeper, more targeted stretches, you can do this exercise, but instead of pulling all your toes at once, you can stretch individual digits.

- You can even switch it up by stretching different combinations of digits. Get creative with this stretch and find what feels good.

Tennis Ball Roll

Plantar fasciitis is inflammation that develops in the fibrous tissue that connects your heel to your foot. This inflammation of the plantar fascia is formed because of the weight that is consistently placed on the foot. The condition can cause pain and immobility. Doing the right stretches can relieve plantar fasciitis to create comfort in the foot so you can move and balance regardless of your activities. For this exercise, you will need a tennis ball, a golf ball, or any firm ball of similar size.

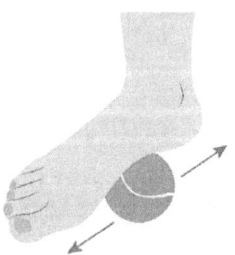

39. Plantar fasciitis is inflammation that develops in the fibrous tissue that connects your heel to your foot. Source: https://images.squarespace-cdn.com/content/v1/574ff940b09f95f3b309b82b/1504482935307-OAFP8SWMG67QTE5IHTZR/tennis-ball-foot-massage.jpg

- While sitting on a chair with one foot flat on the ground, roll your foot along the ball on the floor.

- Adjust the pressure you apply to be as strong or as gentle as you are comfortable with.

- Continue rolling the ball for about three minutes, and then switch feet to repeat the exercise.

- This exercise can be relaxing and stress-relieving because it is like giving yourself a deep tissue massage.

Ankle Circles

Stiff ankles will cause you to limp, so you must do stretches daily to keep them well-oiled and limber. Ankle circles are a simple exercise you can do anywhere.

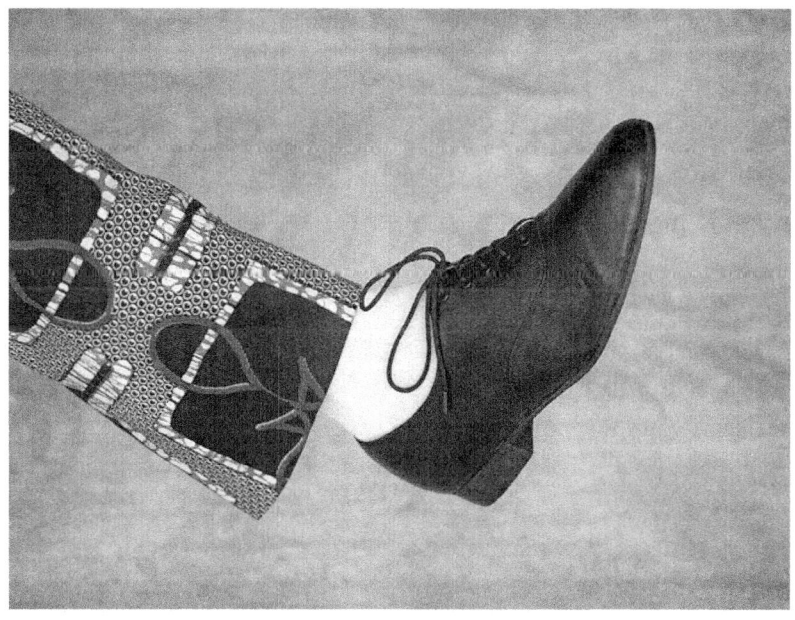

40. Stiff ankles will cause you to limp. Source: https://pixabay.com/photos/foot-shoe-step-footstep-ankle-1744044/

- While sitting up straight in a chair, extend one leg forward or use your arms to lift it off the ground.

- Now rotate your foot ten times clockwise, then rotate it another ten times anti-clockwise.

- After these rotations, bend your foot backward and forward five times.

- Point your toes forward away from your body and hold the stretch for ten seconds, then point your toes toward your knees and hold it for ten seconds.

- Repeat the exercise on your other foot and feel how the tightness in your ankle slowly fades.

Your lower body is the driving force of your mobility. Moving around freely greatly depends on having strong and flexible legs. Knee and ankle pain is common as the joints lose flexibility. Counteracting the stiffness that age brings requires actively stretching daily. When people retire, they often move a lot less because they no longer travel for work. Therefore, doing what is necessary to stay on your feet for decades is crucial. Seated stretches and gentle movements enable you to stay mobile without injuring yourself. Introducing lower body stretches into your daily routine greatly increases your quality of life by keeping you pushing forward.

Chapter 5: Full Body Stretches

The full-body stretches in this chapter are simple and relaxing moves to activate the muscles of the back, chest, calves, arms, quads, and hamstrings. Full body stretches loosen the muscles, improve flexibility, and increase the range of motion. If you do these stretches correctly, your overall physical comfort will be enhanced. Like the stretching exercises in earlier chapters, these exercises enable you to stay agile, alleviate muscle tension, and aid in reducing pain experienced by chronic conditions like osteoarthritis.

These full-body stretching routines can incorporate dynamic or static stretches. Dynamic stretches require controlled movements that stretch a particular group of muscles or joints through a full range of motion. These rhythmic stretches typically mimic your movements during your exercise routine. On the other hand, static stretching requires holding a specific position or posture for fifteen to thirty seconds. While dynamic stretching is usually incorporated into a pre-workout routine, static stretching is done after your exercise routine or workout to relieve muscle tension and relax the body.

Gentle Full-Body Routine

Your gentle-full body stretching routine includes stretching exercises to target every muscle group. Doing a light cardio exercise, like a five-minute walk in the garden, is also recommended to improve blood flow throughout the body. After you finish cardio, start exercises targeting the top of the body and gradually work your way down so you don't miss out on activating any muscle group.

Dynamic Stretching Exercises

Neck Roll

1. Stand up while placing the feet shoulder-width apart.

2. Keep your arms loose and bring your chin close to the chest.

3. Now, rotate your head in an anti-clockwise direction and pause for seven seconds when you have completed one rotation.

4. Repeat the same rotation clockwise and perform at least three rotations in each direction.

Shoulder Roll

1. Stand upright with your feet shoulder-width apart and the arms loose.

2. Keeping the arms straight, slowly raise the shoulders and roll them in a circular motion.

3. Roll the shoulders from back to front and vice versa at least five times to complete the stretching exercise.

Arm Swings

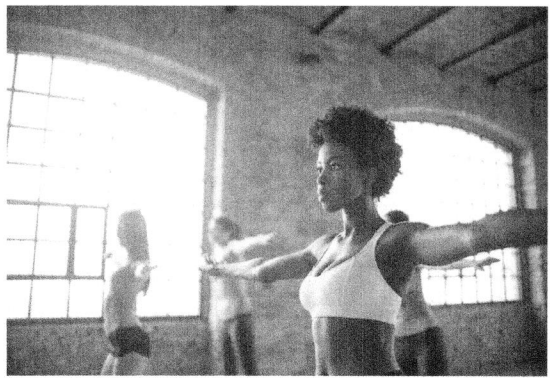

41. *It's important to keep your shoulders relaxed to improve there mobility. https://www.pexels.com/photo/confident-fit-ethnic-woman-training-with-other-sportswomen-in-modern-fitness-studio-3775603/*

1. While keeping your feet shoulder-width apart, extend the arms to shoulder height.

2. Now, swing the arms forward and backward, mimicking a pendulum-like motion.

3. When performing arm swings, keep the shoulders relaxed to improve their mobility.

Leg Swings

1. Perform this exercise while standing upright. You can take the support of a nearby wall to maintain balance.

2. Lift one leg from the ground and swing it back and forth like a pendulum. The other leg must remain firm with the foot in contact with the ground.

3. The hip joint becomes a pivot in this exercise, letting you swing your leg easily.

4. This exercise loosens and warms the hip and thigh muscles, enhancing leg mobility.

High Knees

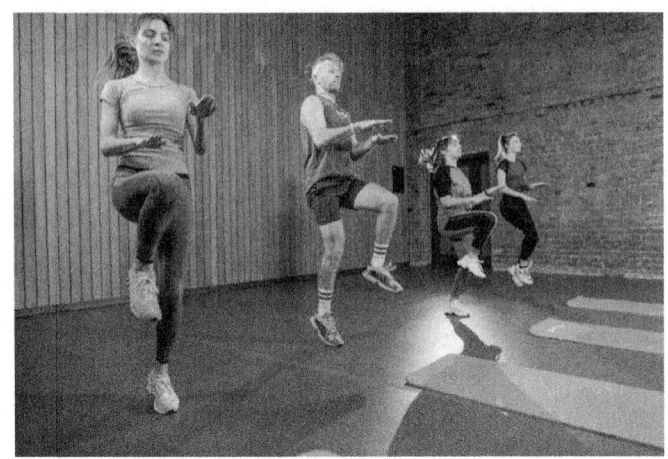

42. Bending the knees boosts the heart rate and decreases the body's core temperature. Source: https://www.pexels.com/photo/a-group-of-people-in-the-fitness-center-6339342/

1. Stand in an upright position with the feet hip-width apart and the arms straight, pointing towards the ground.

2. Bring the left arm forward while keeping it extended. The arm will make a 90-degree angle with the body. As your left arm moves up, bring the right knee up. Repeat the movement on the opposite side and keep the switching between alternate limbs steady for maximum impact.

3. Bending the knees boosts the heart rate, decreases the body's core temperature, and activates quadriceps and hip flexor muscles.

Ankle Circles

1. Sit on a sturdy chair with one leg extended. The chair you pick must be according to your height. However, as a rule of thumb, the exercise chair you pick should be

at a height where your feet can touch the ground and the knees stay bent at right angles.

2. Lift your extended leg off the ground. You must lift the leg at least five inches off the ground.

3. Rotate your ankle in circular motions, clockwise and anti-clockwise.

4. Repeat this ankle circle exercise for both legs.

5. Ankle circles help improve ankle mobility and reduce the risk of lower leg injuries.

Torso Twists

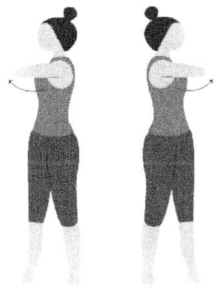

43. Torso twists engage the core muscles and improve spinal mobility. Source: https://d5sbbf6usl3xq.cloudfront.net/trunk_twisting_pose__kati_ shakti_vikasaka_kriya_yoga.png

1. Stand with your feet hip-width apart.

2. Place your hands on your hips or hold the back of a sturdy chair for balance.

3. Gently twist your torso from side to side, mimicking a twisting motion.

4. Keep your feet firmly planted and your movements controlled.

5. Torso twists engage the core muscles and improve spinal mobility.

Leg Swings (Lateral)

1. Stand upright with both hands on the wall

2. While keeping your right leg firm, lift your left leg at least three inches from the ground.

3. Keep the left leg extended and swing it towards the left and then across the body to the right side.

4. Stop the left leg motion as it reaches its original position and switch to the other leg.

This exercise enhances hip mobility and helps loosen the inner and outer thigh muscles.

Hip Circles

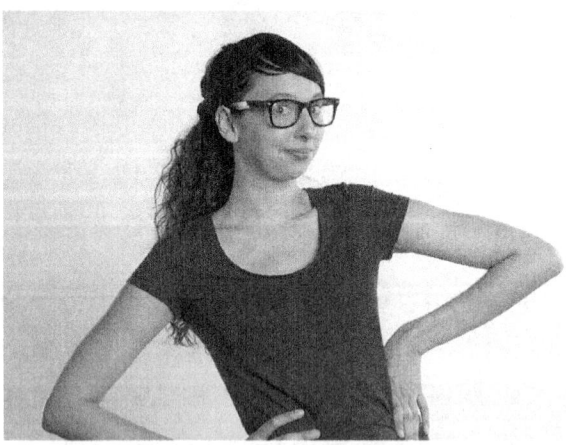

44. Hip circles improve hip joint mobility and flexibility. Source: https://pixabay.com/photos/woman-young-pretty-fashion-sexy-3355952/

1. Stand with your feet hip-width apart.

2. Place your hands on your hips.

3. Gently make circular motions with your hips, rotating them in clockwise and anti-clockwise directions.

4. Hip circles improve hip joint mobility and flexibility.

Shoulder Circles

1. Stand with your feet shoulder-width apart.

2. Extend your arms to the sides so they become parallel to the floor.

3. Make circular motions with your shoulders, rolling them forward and backward.

4. Shoulder circles warm up the shoulder joints and upper body.

March in Place with Arm Crosses

1. March in place, lifting your knees slightly.

2. As you march, cross, and open your arms in front of your chest.

3. This exercise simultaneously engages the lower and upper body while improving circulation.

Knee to Chest March

1. Stand with your feet hip-width apart.

2. Lift one knee toward your chest, holding it with both hands.

3. March in place, alternating between each leg.

4. This exercise stretches the hip flexors and improves balance.

Static Stretching Exercises

Neck Stretch

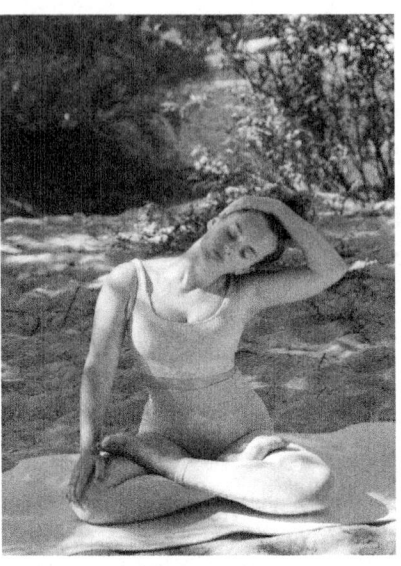

45. The neck stretch releases tension in the neck and shoulders. Source: https://www.pexels.com/photo/a-woman-in-activewear-stretching-her-neck-8534776/

1. Sit or stand with your back straight.

2. Tilt your head to one side, bringing your ear toward your shoulder.

3. Hold this position for 15-30 seconds while feeling a gentle stretch along the side of your neck.

4. Repeat the stretch on the other side.

5. The neck stretch releases tension in the neck and shoulders.

Shoulder and Arm Stretch

1. Keeping the back straight, sit on a chair or stand upright.

2. Lift one arm to the shoulder height and bring it across your chest.

3. Using the opposite hand, gently push the extended arm closer to the chest, feeling a stretch in the shoulder and the arm.

4. Hold for 15 to 30 seconds and repeat two to four times for each arm.

Chest Opener

1. Stand with your feet hip-width apart.

2. Clasp your hands behind your back.

3. Straighten your arms and gently lift them while squeezing your shoulder blades together.

4. Hold for 15-30 seconds.

5. The chest opener stretches the chest and shoulders, improving posture.

Hamstring Stretch

1. Sit on the edge of the exercise-like chair while keeping the spine straight. You'll be sitting in a forward-leaning position. Extend one leg out while keeping the knee and toes straight.

2. Gently stretch the corresponding arm out and reach toward your toes, keeping your back straight.

3. Hold for 15-30 seconds on each leg.

4. This exercise increases flexibility in the hamstring muscles.

Quadriceps Stretch

1. Stand beside a sturdy chair for balance.

2. Bend the knee of the outside leg and bring your heel toward your buttocks.

3. Gently hold your ankle with your hand to feel the stretch in the front of your thigh.

4. Turn around and repeat for the other side

5. Hold for 15-30 seconds on each leg.

6. The quadriceps stretch targets the front thigh muscles.

Calf Stretch

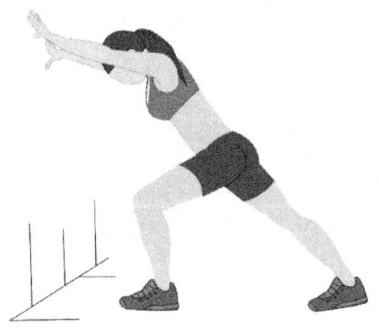

46. This stretch improves calf muscle flexibility. Source: https://www.spotebi.com/wp-content/uploads/2015/03/calf-stretch-exercise-illustration.jpg

1. Stand straight with both hands on the wall. Your feet must be hip-width apart.

2. Step one foot back, keeping it straight.

3. Gentle press the heel of the back foot into the floor.

4. Hold for 15-30 seconds on each leg.

5. This stretch improves calf muscle flexibility.

Hip Flexor Stretch

1. Slide the left foot back so the left knee comes closer to the floor. The right knee should now be below the right hip. Keep the left foot on the ground for support.

2. Slide the left foot back so the left knee comes closer to the floor. The right knee should now be below the right hip. Keep the left foot on the ground for support.

3. Tighten the buttocks and hold for at least 30 seconds. Repeat with each leg.

4. The hip flexor stretch targets the hip flexor and quadriceps muscles.

Spine Twist

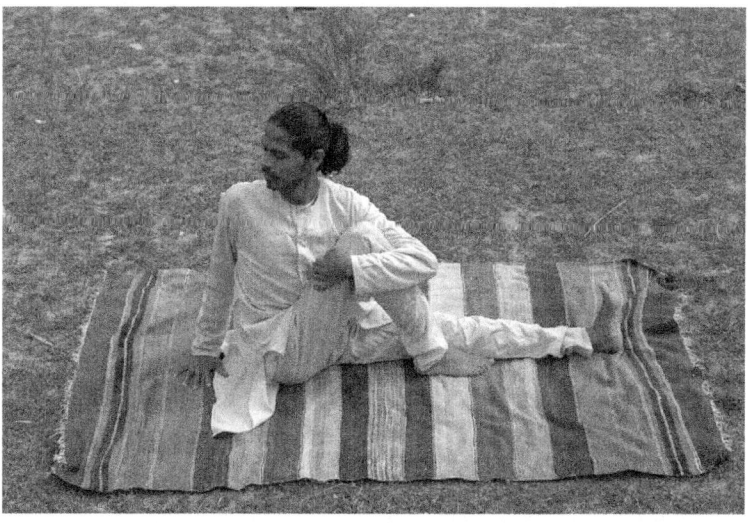

47. The spine twist enhances spinal mobility and stretches the oblique muscles. Source: https://pixabay.com/photos/spine-twist-pose-yoga-yogi-indian-2653576/

1. Sit in a chair with your feet flat on the floor.

2. Gently twist your upper body to one side while keeping your hips facing forward.

3. Hold for 15-30 seconds on each side.

4. The spine twist enhances spinal mobility and stretches the oblique muscles.

Full Body Stretch

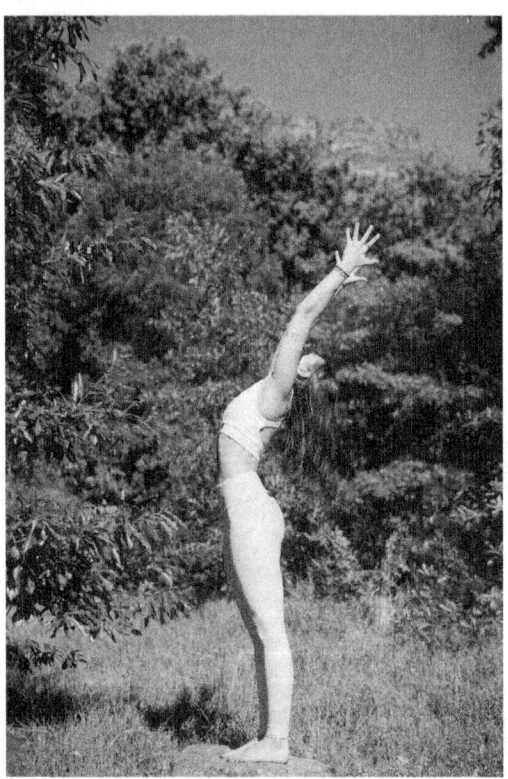

48. This exercise provides a full-body stretch, lengthening the entire body. Source: https://www.pexels.com/photo/woman-in-white-tank-top-raising-her-hands-3820430/

1. Stand with your feet shoulder-width apart.

2. Reach your arms overhead and stretch upward, rising onto your toes to add a calf stretch.

3. Hold for 15-30 seconds.

4. This exercise provides a full-body stretch, lengthening the entire body.

Seated Trunk Twist

1. Sit on a chair with your feet flat on the floor. The feet must be hip-width apart.

2. Place your right hand on your left knee.

3. Gently twist your upper body to the left, keeping your hips facing forward.

4. Hold for 15-30 seconds and repeat on the other side.

5. The seated trunk twist stretches the spine and oblique muscles.

Seated Butterfly Stretch

1. Sit on the edge of a chair with your knees at 90 degrees and your feet on the ground.

2. Bring the soles of your feet together, allowing your knees to fall to the sides.

3. Gently press your knees down with your hands.

4. Hold for 15-30 seconds.

5. The seated butterfly stretch stretches the inner thighs.

Seated Heel-to-Toe Stretch

1. Sit on the edge of a chair in a normal sitting position where your feet are on the ground, and the knee makes a 90-degree angle.

2. Extend one leg straight out and flex your foot.

3. Gently reach forward, trying to touch your toes.

4. Hold for 15-30 seconds on each leg.

5. This exercise stretches the hamstrings and calves.

Ankle Flexion and Extension

1. Sit on a chair with your feet hip-width apart, flat on the floor.

2. Lift one foot off the ground at least three inches above the ground.

3. Flex and point your foot, alternating between these movements.

4. Perform this exercise for both feet.

5. Ankle flexion and extension improve ankle mobility and help prevent stiffness.

Seated Shoulder Stretch

1. Sit on a chair with your back straight.

2. Extend one arm across your chest.

3. Use your opposite hand to press your arm closer to your chest gently.

4. Hold for 15-30 seconds one each arm.

5. The seated shoulder stretch releases tension in the shoulders and upper back.

Neck Side Stretch

1. Sit comfortably in the chair with the feet hip-width apart

2. Bring the right hand behind your back and place the left hand on top of the head.

3. Now, gently tilt the head to the left and hold it for at least ten seconds.

4. Repeat the exercise for the other side and perform at least two to four repetitions.

5. The neck side stretch activates the trapezius and strengths the neck muscles.

These full-body stretching exercises may seem daunting, especially for seniors who are not physically active. However, performing a full body stretching routine takes only ten to twenty minutes, priming the body for more physically demanding exercises.

Yoga-Inspired Stretches

Yoga-inspired stretches combine the principles of yoga with traditional stretching exercises to improve flexibility, balance, and overall well-being. These stretches focus on physical and mental well-being, making them well-suited for seniors. Here are detailed yoga-inspired stretches for seniors:

Child's Pose

1. Start on your hands and knees.

2. Sit back on your heels, with your knees hip-width and big toes touching each other.

3. Extend your arms forward while the palms remain in contact with the ground and relax your forehead on the floor.

4. Hold for 30 seconds to 1 minute, focusing on deep breaths to release tension and promote relaxation.

Downward-Facing Dog

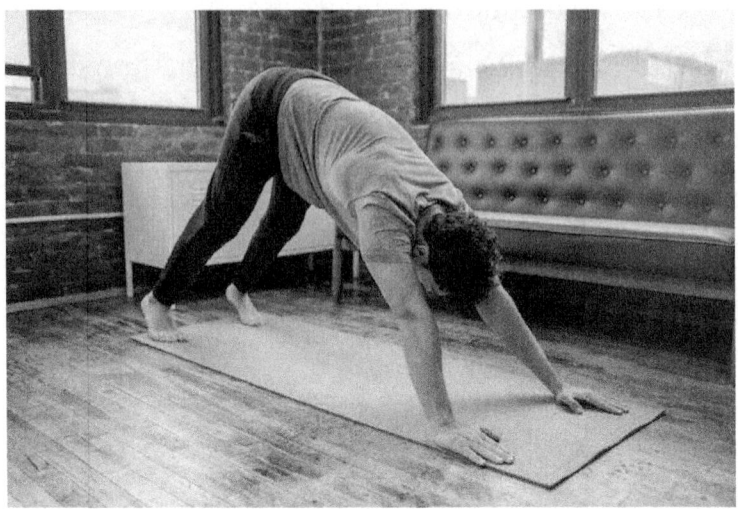

49. This stretch improves flexibility in the back, shoulders, and hamstrings. Source: https://www.pexels.com/photo/man-doing-yoga-in-downward-facing-dog-pose-on-mat-6303796/

1. Begin with your hands and knees touching the ground. You should position yourself so that the knees come underneath the hips and the wrists underneath the shoulders.

2. Tuck the toes under and push through the knees, lifting your hips and straightening your legs, forming an inverted V-shape.

3. Press your palms into the mat and keep your heels down (it's okay if they don't touch the floor).

4. This stretch improves flexibility in the back, shoulders, and hamstrings.

Triangle Pose

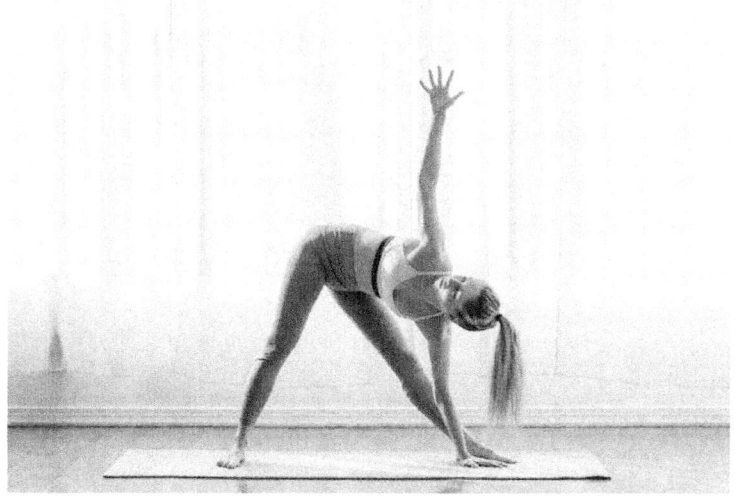

50. Triangle Pose stretches the hamstrings, hips, and sides of the body. Source: https://www.pexels.com/photo/woman-doing-yoga-in-triangle-pose-6454064/

1. Stand with your feet about 3-4 feet apart.

2. Turn your right foot out 90 degrees and your left foot slightly inward.

3. Extend your arms to the sides at shoulder height.

4. Bend at your right hip and reach your right hand down to your shin or a block.

5. Extend your left arm up toward the ceiling.

6. Hold for 30 seconds to 1 minute, then switch sides.

7. Triangle Pose stretches the hamstrings, hips, and sides of the body.

Seated Forward Bend

1. Keep the feet straight and the legs extended in a natural position.

2. Inhale, lengthen your spine, and exhale, gently fold forward from your hips.

3. Reach for your shins, ankles, or feet, depending on your flexibility.

4. Hold for 30 seconds to 1 minute, focusing on deep breaths.

5. This stretch improves hamstring flexibility and calms the mind.

Pigeon Pose

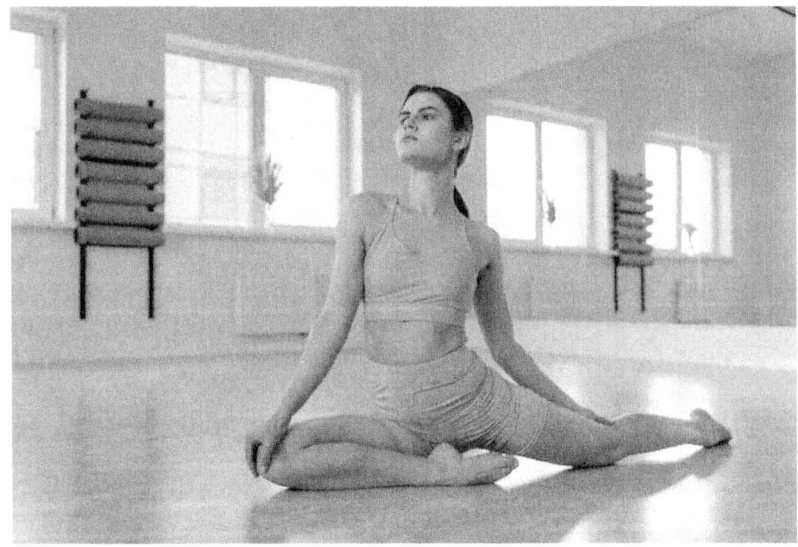

51. You'll need to start this exercise by doing a yoga pose. Source: https://www.pexels.com/photo/a-young-woman-in-a-half-pigeon-yoga-pose-7318689/

1. You'll need to start this exercise by doing a yoga pose. The tabletop position is the starting point for many yoga exercises. You can make this position by bringing your knees and hands to touch the ground. The hips should be above the knees and the shoulders directly above the elbow.

2. Slide your left leg straight back, keeping your hips square.

3. Fold forward over your front leg and rest on your forearms or forehead.

4. Hold for 30 seconds to 1 minute, then switch sides.

5. Pigeon Pose opens the hips and increases flexibility in the groin area.

Tree Pose

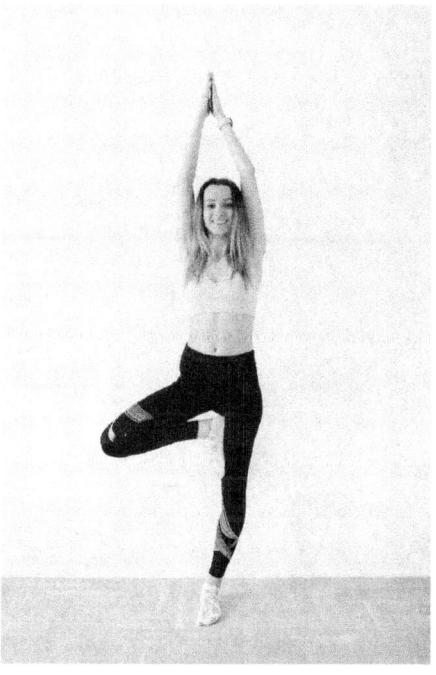

52. Tree Pose enhances balance and strengthens the legs. Source: https://www.pexels.com/photo/cheerful-sportswoman-practicing-yoga-tree-pose-4498150/

1. Stand with your feet hip-width apart.

2. Shift your weight onto your right foot and place the sole of your left foot on your inner right thigh or calf.

3. Keep your hands at your heart center or raise them overhead.

4. Hold for 30 seconds to 1 minute, then switch legs.

5. Tree Pose enhances balance and strengthens the legs.

Warrior I

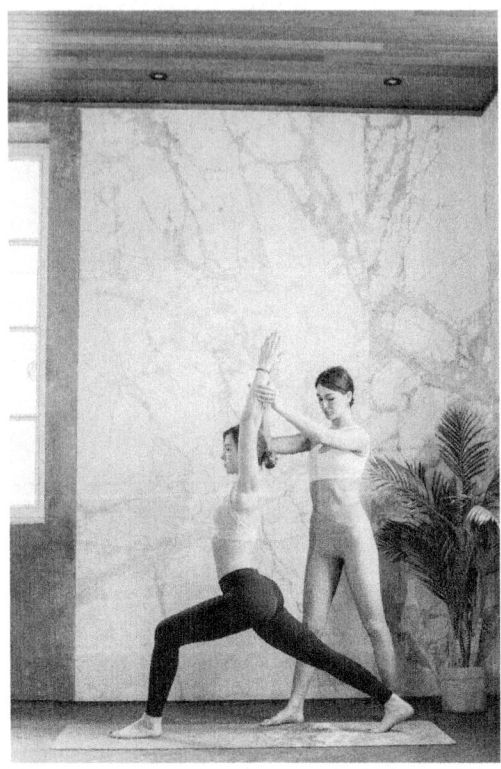

53. Warrior I stretches the hips and legs and strengthens the lower body. Source: https://www.pexels.com/photo/yoga-instructor-helping-a-student-3822691/

1. Stand with your feet about 3-4 feet apart.

2. Turn your right foot out 90 degrees and your left foot slightly inward.

3. Bend your right knee and square your hips toward the front.

4. Raise your arms overhead, keeping them shoulder-width apart.

5. Hold for 30 seconds to 1 minute, then switch sides.

6. Warrior I stretches the hips and legs and strengthens the lower body.

Warrior II

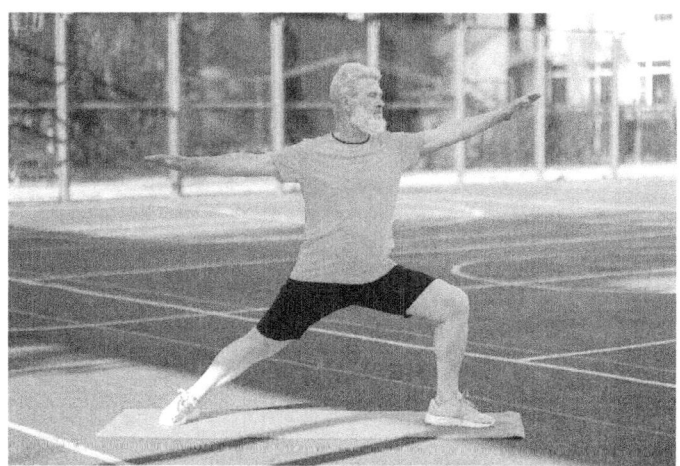

54. Warrior II stretches the hips and inner thighs and enhances focus and balance. Source: https://www.pexels.com/photo/senior-man-in-orange-shirt-and-black pants doing yoga-5067957/

1. Start with your feet about 3-4 feet apart.

2. Turn your right foot out 90 degrees and your left foot slightly inward.

3. Extend your arms to the sides at shoulder height.

4. Bend your right knee while keeping your hips square to the side.

5. Gaze over your right hand.

6. Hold for 30 seconds to 1 minute, then switch sides.

7. Warrior II stretches the hips and inner thighs and enhances focus and balance.

Bridge Pose

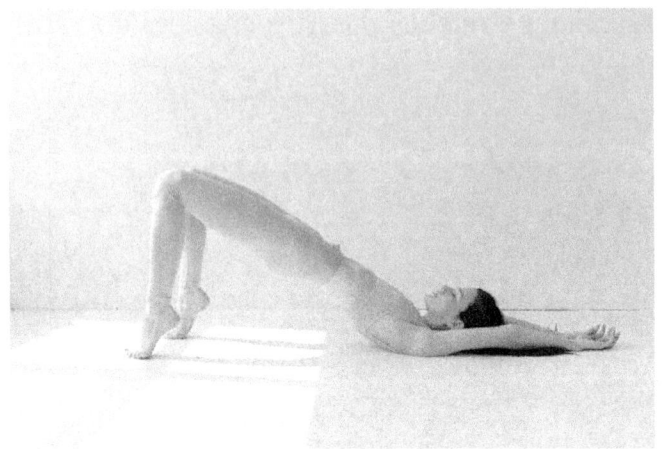

55. Bridge Pose stretches the chest, neck, and spine while strengthening the back and legs. Source: https://www.pexels.com/photo/graceful-woman-performing-variation-of-setu-bandha-sarvangasana-yoga-pose-5012071/

1. Lie on your back with your knees bent and feet flat on the floor, hip-width apart.

2. Place your arms by your sides, palms down.

3. Lift your hips off the ground while pressing into your feet and arms.

4. Keep your neck relaxed and shoulders on the mat.

5. Hold for 30 seconds to 1 minute.

6. Bridge Pose stretches the chest, neck, and spine while strengthening the back and legs.

Seated Twist

1. Sit with your legs extended in front of you and your feet flexed.

2. Bend your right knee and place your right foot on the outside of your left thigh.

3. Place your left hand on your right knee and your right hand behind you.

4. Inhale to lengthen your spine, and exhale to twist to the right.

5. Hold for 30 seconds to 1 minute, then switch sides.

6. Seated twists improve spinal mobility and digestion.

Extended Puppy Pose

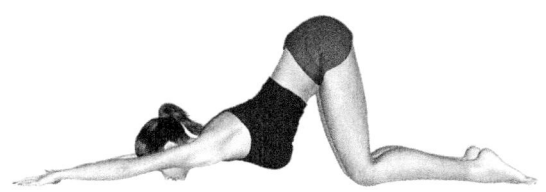

56. Extended Puppy Pose stretches the spine, shoulders, and arms. Source: https://pixabay.com/illustrations/yoga-girl-fitness-pose-heath-7120612/

1. Start on your hands and knees.

2. Walk your hands forward while lowering your chest toward the mat.

3. Keep your hips above your knees.

4. Extend your arms and stretch your spine forward.

5. Hold for 30 seconds to 1 minute.

6. Extended Puppy Pose stretches the spine, shoulders, and arms.

These yoga-inspired stretches suit seniors and provide a holistic approach to improving physical and mental well-being. As with any exercise, it's essential to perform them with mindfulness, focusing on deep, controlled breaths and listening to your body's limits to avoid strain or injury. Yoga-inspired stretches can enhance flexibility, balance, and relaxation, making them a valuable addition to a senior's fitness routine.

Tai Chi for Flexibility

Tai chi is a gentle and effective practice for seniors to improve their flexibility. It incorporates slow, flowing movements and emphasizes balance and mindfulness. Tai chi gradually stretches and lengthens muscles, tendons, and ligaments throughout the body through these gentle stretching movements.

The focus on the mind-body connection allows practitioners to identify areas of tension and stiffness, making it easier to address these issues and gradually increase flexibility. Furthermore, tai chi's slow, controlled movements lubricate the joints, reducing joint stiffness and improving their mobility, which is especially beneficial for maintaining joint health as you age. In addition to enhancing physical flexibility, tai chi strengthens the muscles around the joints and improves balance, reducing the risk of falls and injuries. Its adaptability to different fitness levels allows for gradual progression and safe practice. The practice's relaxation techniques and deep breathing also help reduce stress, making it easier for the body to stretch and improve flexibility.

Tai chi offers a holistic approach to enhancing flexibility, combining physical, mental, and emotional well-being, and provides long-term benefits for seniors. However, you must take classes from a certified tai chi instructor to develop your mind and body connection and suggest the right exercises for your age group and fitness.

Here are some basic tai chi practices you can do at home.

Deep Breathing

1. Find a quiet, comfortable space to sit or stand with good posture.

2. Close your eyes and start taking slow, deep breaths.

3. Inhale deeply through your nose, expanding your abdomen rather than your chest.

4. Exhale slowly through your mouth, letting go of tension and stress with each breath.

5. Focus on the rise and fall of your abdomen with each breath, and let your mind clear as you continue to breathe deeply.

Body Scan

1. Begin by standing or sitting comfortably with your eyes closed.

2. Mentally scan your body from head to toe, one part at a time.

3. Pay attention to areas of tension, discomfort, or stress you notice as you go.

4. Consciously release the tension in each area as you progress, imagining it melting away with your breath.

5. Continue to breathe deeply and with mindfulness as you scan your body, releasing tension and promoting relaxation.

Progressive Muscle Relaxation

1. Find a quiet and comfortable spot to sit or lie down.

2. Start at your toes and work your way up through your body or start at the head and work down your body.

3. Tense each muscle group for a few seconds and then release.

4. Focus on the sensations of tension and relaxation, allowing your muscles to unwind.

5. By systematically releasing tension in this way, you encourage deep relaxation throughout your body.

Guided Meditation

1. Find a calm and quiet place where you won't be disturbed.

2. Listen to a guided meditation or visualization recording that walks you through relaxation techniques.

3. Follow the guidance, which may include deep breathing, visualization, and progressive relaxation.

4. These recordings often help you focus on relaxation and reduce stress with the soothing voice and imagery provided.

Tai Chi Flow

1. Practice a simplified tai chi sequence or a few of your favorite tai chi movements.

2. Concentrate on the slow, flowing motions and coordinate them with deep, rhythmic breathing.

3. Visualize the movements as a way to release tension and enhance flexibility.

4. Pay close attention to the connection between your breath and the fluid movements, allowing them to work together for relaxation.

Mindfulness Meditation

1. Sit comfortably in a quiet space.

2. Focus your attention on your breath as it naturally flows in and out.

3. When your mind wanders to other thoughts, without judgment, gently redirect your focus back to your breath.

4. Engage in mindfulness by observing your thoughts and feelings without judgment, letting them come and go as you return your focus to your breath.

Relaxing Music

1. Create a calming atmosphere by playing soft, soothing music or nature sounds in the background.

2. This music can set the tone for relaxation and provide a soothing auditory backdrop for your other relaxation practices.

Visualization

1. Find a comfortable place to sit or lie down with your eyes closed.

2. Visualize yourself in a peaceful and relaxing location, like a tranquil garden, a serene beach, or a peaceful forest.

3. Imagine the sights, sounds, and sensations of that place in vivid detail, focusing on the sense of relaxation and peace it brings.

Self-Massage

1. Use gentle self-massage techniques on tension areas like your neck, shoulders, and back.

2. Use your fingers or the palms of your hands to knead or stroke these areas gently, releasing muscle tension and promoting relaxation.

Warm Beverage Ritual

1. Brew a cup of soothing herbal tea or warm water with a squeeze of lemon.

2. Sit in a quiet and comfortable spot.

3. Sip your tea or warm beverage slowly, savoring each sip and paying attention to the warmth and relaxation it provides.

4. The process of making and enjoying a warm beverage can become a comforting and grounding ritual promoting relaxation.

Practicing these tai chii-inspired relaxation techniques can reduce stress, enhance flexibility, and promote overall well-being in the comfort of your home. Regular practice, even just a few minutes each day, can significantly reduce stress and increase relaxation and flexibility.

Chapter 6: Stretching for Specific Conditions

Stretching can be crucial in managing pain and conditions like arthritis and osteoporosis in seniors. For arthritis, gentle and regular stretching exercises can help improve joint flexibility and reduce stiffness, alleviating pain and improving overall joint function. Stretching also helps maintain a healthy range of motion, making everyday activities more accessible for seniors with arthritis.

Specific weight-bearing and balance-focused stretches can be particularly beneficial for osteoporosis. Weight-bearing exercises, like standing stretches, can help stimulate bone growth and increase bone density, which is crucial for seniors with reduced bone strength. Balance-focused stretches enhance stability and reduce the risk of falls, which is essential for individuals with osteoporosis, as they are more prone to fractures.

However, seniors with these conditions must consult a healthcare professional or a physical therapist before starting a stretching regimen. They can create a tailored stretching program that is safe and effective, considering the individual's specific condition and needs. When done correctly, regular stretching can be a valuable part of a senior's overall wellness plan to manage arthritis and osteoporosis. Here's everything you need to know about stretching and how to use it effectively to manage these medical conditions for a healthier and pain-free life.

Stretching for Arthritis Relief

Understanding Arthritis

Arthritis is a chronic condition affecting the joints, leading to symptoms like pain, swelling, and stiffness. There are several types of arthritis, with osteoarthritis and rheumatoid arthritis being the most common. Arthritis often limits joint mobility, making it challenging for individuals to perform daily tasks and engage in physical activities.

Types of Arthritis

Beyond osteoarthritis and rheumatoid arthritis, other common types include gout, ankylosing spondylitis, and psoriatic arthritis. Each type might require a tailored approach to stretching and pain management.

Localized Pain

Arthritis can affect specific joints or multiple joints throughout the body. Identifying the specific joints involved is essential as this can determine the most effective stretching exercises for you.

Arthritis Flare-Ups

Arthritis symptoms come and go in episodes known as flare-ups. During flare-ups, it's advisable to temporarily modify or reduce the intensity of your stretching routine to avoid exacerbating pain.

The Benefits of Stretching for Arthritis Relief

Stretching can be a highly effective approach to arthritis management because it addresses several key aspects of the condition.

Improved Joint Flexibility

Stretching exercises help maintain or improve the range of motion in your joints. For individuals with arthritis, this is crucial as it prevents joint stiffness and allows more natural movement.

Muscle Tension Reduction

Stretching reduces muscle tension around affected joints, indirectly alleviating pressure on the joints and reducing pain and discomfort.

Increased Circulation

Stretching can improve blood flow to the joints and surrounding tissues. Enhanced circulation promotes healing and decreases inflammation.

Enhanced Strength and Stability

Proper stretching can help strengthen the muscles supporting your joints, improving overall joint stability and function.

Stretching can reduce pain by releasing tension and promoting blood flow. This, in turn, helps decrease inflammation in and around affected joints.

Functional Improvement

Improved joint flexibility and muscle strength can lead to increased functionality in everyday activities. It can make it easier to perform tasks like walking, climbing stairs, and reaching overhead.

Quality of Life

Arthritis often impacts an individual's quality of life. By incorporating stretching into your daily routine, you can experience a significant improvement in your overall well-being, both physically and emotionally.

Types of Stretches for Arthritis Relief

Range of Motion Exercises

These gentle, repetitive movements aim to maintain or improve the full range of motion in your joints. Some common examples include wrist circles, shoulder rolls, ankle circles, and knee bends.

Tailor your stretching routine to address the specific joints affected by arthritis. For instance, if your knee joints are affected, focus on quadriceps and hamstring stretches. If it's your hands, incorporate finger and wrist stretches.

Range of Motion Devices

In some cases, especially with severe arthritis, healthcare professionals might recommend using a range of motion devices, like splints or braces, to assist in stretching and maintaining joint flexibility.

Progressive Stretching

Gradually increase the intensity and duration of your stretches as your body becomes more accustomed to the exercises. Start with easier stretches and gradually move to more advanced ones.

Morning Stretching

Many arthritis patients find it beneficial to perform gentle stretching exercises in the morning to alleviate stiffness and improve mobility throughout the day.

Static Stretching

This involves holding a specific stretch position for a set period. It targets specific muscles and helps alleviate muscle tension around the joints. For instance, you can perform calf stretches, quadriceps stretches, and hamstring stretches.

Dynamic Stretching

Dynamic stretches use controlled, repetitive movements to prepare your muscles and joints for physical activity. Leg swings, arm circles, and torso twists are examples of dynamic stretches.

Yoga and Tai Chi

These mind-body practices incorporate a wide range of stretching exercises, often with a focus on breath control and meditation. They improve flexibility, balance, and overall well-being, making them valuable for arthritis management.

Water-Based Exercise

Aquatic exercise in a pool provides a supportive, low-impact environment for stretching and strengthening. Water aerobics and water walking are effective for individuals with arthritis as the buoyancy of water reduces joint strain.

Breathing and Relaxation Techniques

Stress management is crucial for arthritis patients, as stress can exacerbate symptoms. Deep breathing exercises and meditation can be integrated into your routine to reduce tension and promote calm.

Additional Tips

Warm-Up

Before stretching, perform a gentle warm-up, like walking or riding a stationary bike for a few minutes, to increase blood flow and prepare your muscles and joints for stretching.

Balance

Focus on stretching both sides of your body equally to maintain balance and symmetry.

Professional Guidance

Consult a physical therapist or occupational therapist with expertise in arthritis management. They can assess your condition and create a personalized stretching program to ensure your safety and effectiveness.

Pain Assessment

Pay close attention to your body. If you experience increased pain or discomfort during or after stretching, consult your healthcare provider to adjust your routine or explore other treatment options.

Consistency

Commit to a daily stretching routine. Regularity is essential for achieving and maintaining the benefits. Consult your healthcare provider about the best time to stretch if you're on medication for arthritis. Some medications could affect muscle or joint function, so coordinating your stretching routine with your medication schedule is important.

Heat and Cold

Applying heat or cold therapy before or after stretching can help reduce inflammation and improve your stretching routine's effectiveness.

Adaptive Equipment

Consider using adaptive equipment, like resistance bands or props, to make stretching easier and more effective, especially if arthritis has limited your range of motion.

Hydration

Staying hydrated is essential for maintaining joint health. Dehydration can exacerbate joint discomfort, so ensure you drink enough water throughout the day.

Nutrition

A balanced diet with anti-inflammatory foods, such as fish rich in omega-3 fatty acids and plenty of fruits and vegetables, can complement your stretching routine and help manage arthritis symptoms.

Supportive Footwear

Properly fitting and supportive footwear can help alleviate pressure on arthritic joints in the lower extremities. Invest in shoes that provide cushioning and stability.

Regular Check-Ups

Continue to have regular check-ups with your healthcare provider to monitor your arthritis, adjust your treatment plan as necessary, and ensure your stretching regimen aligns with your overall care for improved flexibility and reduced pain.

While stretching is a valuable component of arthritis management, it should be part of a comprehensive treatment plan, including medication, lifestyle adjustments, and, in some cases, surgery. Always work closely with your healthcare provider to determine the most suitable approach for your specific arthritis type and severity.

Stretching for Osteoporosis Prevention

Understanding Osteoporosis

Bone Structure

Osteoporosis

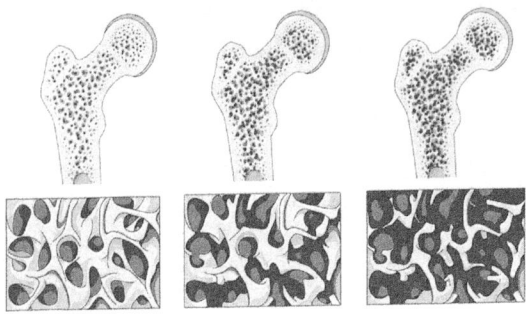

57. Osteoporosis affects the density and quality of bones. Source: Laboratoires Servier, CC BY-SA 3.0 <https://creativecommons.org/licenses/by-sa/3.0>, via Wikimedia Commons: https://commons.wikimedia.org/wiki/File:Osteoporosis_-- _Smart-Servier.jpg

Osteoporosis affects the density and quality of bones, causing them to become porous and fragile. Understanding that bones are living tissue that constantly remodels is important. Osteoporosis occurs when the balance between bone formation and bone resorption is disrupted.

Risk Factors

In addition to postmenopausal women, family history, and a sedentary lifestyle, other risk factors for osteoporosis include low body weight, smoking, excessive alcohol consumption, and certain medications (like corticosteroids). There are also specific medical conditions that affect calcium absorption.

Fracture Risk

Osteoporosis significantly increases the risk of fractures, particularly in weight-bearing bones like the hip, spine, and wrist. Fractures in the spine can lead to loss of height and poor posture.

The Benefits of Stretching for Osteoporosis Prevention

Improved Balance and Fall Prevention

Stretching exercises focusing on balance can help prevent falls. Since individuals with osteoporosis are more prone to fractures from even minor falls, enhanced balance is crucial for reducing the risk of injury.

Enhanced Flexibility and Range of Motion

Stretching increases joint flexibility, making it easier to perform daily activities without straining your bones and muscles. Improved range of motion can also prevent discomfort or pain associated with stiff joints.

Stimulating Bone Growth

Weight-bearing stretches stimulate bone growth and increase bone density, which is essential for preventing further bone loss and maintaining overall bone health.

Types of Stretches for Osteoporosis Prevention

Weight-Bearing Stretches

Include standing leg lifts, calf raises, lunges, and squats in your stretching routine. These exercises place mechanical stress on your bones, stimulating bone formation and maintenance.

Balance Exercises

Balance-focused stretches, like standing on one leg, tree pose in yoga or heel-to-toe walking, improve your stability. Strengthening your core muscles is also essential for balance.

Core Strengthening

A strong core, including your abdominal and back muscles, is essential for maintaining proper posture and spinal stability, reducing the risk of fractures in the spine. Incorporate core-strengthening exercises like planks and bridges.

Pilates and Tai Chi

These exercise methods are particularly effective for osteoporosis prevention. They emphasize posture, balance, and core strength, promoting bone health.

Resistance Bands

Using resistance bands in your stretching routine can add a strength component to your workout, helping build muscle mass and support bone health.

Additional Tips

Consult a Healthcare Professional

Before starting a stretching or exercise routine, consult with a healthcare provider or physical therapist who can assess your bone density and overall physical condition. They can help you create a personalized and safe stretching plan.

Proper Technique

Ensure that you use proper technique during stretching exercises. Perform each stretch slowly and avoid sudden jerking movements to prevent muscle or joint strains.

Comprehensive Exercise

While stretching is beneficial, it should be part of a comprehensive exercise program. Incorporate weight-bearing activities like walking, hiking, or dancing and resistance training to improve muscle support around your bones.

Nutrition

Maintain a diet rich in calcium and vitamin D, as these are essential for bone health. Dairy products, leafy greens, fortified foods, and supplements, if necessary, can help ensure that you get the desired nutrients for your bones.

Hydration

Stay well-hydrated, as dehydration can affect your bones. Proper hydration ensures the effective transport of nutrients to your bones.

Posture Awareness

Good posture is essential for reducing stress on your spine and minimizing the risk of spinal fractures. Ergonomic adjustments in daily activities and ergonomic aids can also help.

Fall Prevention

Take steps to prevent falls, like removing tripping hazards, using handrails on stairs, and considering balance and strength training to improve stability.

Regular Monitoring

Regular bone density tests, as recommended by your healthcare provider, can help you track changes in bone health. If necessary, adjustments to your prevention strategy can be made.

Always seek professional guidance, especially if you have osteoporosis, to ensure that your stretching regimen aligns with your specific needs and health status.

Managing Chronic Pain through Stretching

Understanding Chronic Pain

Chronic pain is often defined as pain that lasts for more than 12 weeks, extending beyond the typical period of healing for an injury or illness. It is not merely a physical sensation but also an emotional and psychological experience that profoundly affects a person's life.

Types of Chronic Pain

Chronic pain can manifest in various ways. Neuropathic pain results from nerve damage or dysfunction, including shooting, burning, or tingling sensations. In contrast, musculoskeletal pain is from muscle or joint issues and is characterized by aching stiffness or cramping.

Centralized Pain Syndromes

Conditions like fibromyalgia, where pain is widespread, are often accompanied by fatigue and sleep disturbances.

Causes of Chronic Pain

Chronic pain can have many underlying causes, and understanding these factors is crucial for effective pain management. One common cause is injury, where pain persists long after the initial injury has healed, often due to residual tissue damage or nerve changes.

Inflammatory conditions like arthritis or autoimmune diseases can lead to persistent pain, with inflammation in the joints and surrounding tissues causing discomfort and stiffness. Whether from injuries, diseases, or conditions like diabetes, nerve damage can result in chronic neuropathic pain characterized by sensations like burning or stabbing. Musculoskeletal issues, such as fibromyalgia or chronic back pain, involve abnormalities in muscles and soft tissues, leading to chronic discomfort.

Additionally, degenerative diseases like osteoarthritis cause gradual joint and bone deterioration, resulting in long-lasting pain. Psychological factors, like stress, anxiety, or depression, can exacerbate chronic pain, emphasizing the interconnection between emotional well-being and pain.

Centralized pain syndromes like fibromyalgia impact the central nervous system, causing widespread pain and sensitivity. Post-surgical pain can also lead to chronic discomfort stemming from nerve damage, scar tissue, or surgical complications.

Chronic pain can be a symptom of underlying health conditions like cancer, multiple sclerosis, or complex regional pain syndrome (CRPS). Lifestyle factors, including poor posture, obesity, and muscle overuse, contribute to chronic pain, especially in the back, neck, and joints. In some instances, genetic factors make individuals more susceptible to certain chronic pain conditions.

Recognizing that chronic pain is often multifaceted, with multiple contributing elements, is essential. Effectively managing chronic pain requires a comprehensive evaluation by a healthcare professional to identify the underlying causes and develop a personalized treatment plan that includes stretching, medications, physical therapy, and lifestyle adjustments. The aim is to address the physical and emotional aspects of pain for improved quality of life and pain relief.

The Benefits of Stretching for Chronic Pain Management

Pain Reduction

Stretching helps relieve chronic pain by promoting the release of endorphins, the body's natural painkillers, and reducing muscle tension often associated with pain.

Improved Flexibility

Stretching exercises enhance joint flexibility and increase your range of motion, reducing the risk of muscle strains and pain caused by stiffness.

Muscle Relaxation

Muscle spasms and tightness are common sources of chronic pain. Stretching promotes muscle relaxation, reducing discomfort and pain.

Enhanced Blood Flow

Stretching encourages blood flow to the muscles, delivering essential nutrients and oxygen. Improved circulation can assist in pain relief and tissue healing.

Stress Reduction

Chronic pain often leads to emotional stress and anxiety. Incorporating deep breathing and relaxation techniques with stretching can reduce stress, improve mood, and contribute to overall well-being.

Types of Stretches for Chronic Pain Management

Dynamic Stretches

Dynamic stretching involves controlled, repetitive movements, taking your body through a range of motion gently. These are excellent warm-up exercises, as they prepare your muscles and joints for more intense activities.

Static Stretches

Static stretching consists of holding specific positions for a set duration. These stretches target individual muscle groups and effectively increase flexibility and reduce muscle tension.

Yoga and Pilates

Yoga and Pilates combine stretching, strength, and flexibility exercises, emphasizing mindfulness and relaxation.

These practices are beneficial for chronic pain management due to their holistic approach.

Water-Based Exercise

Water-based exercises in a pool provide a low-impact environment that's gentle on the body. The buoyancy of water reduces strain, making it ideal for individuals with chronic pain. Water aerobics and swimming offer stretching and strengthening benefits.

Breathing and Relaxation Techniques

Deep breathing exercises, meditation, guided imagery, and progressive muscle relaxation can complement stretching to manage the emotional aspects of chronic pain. These techniques reduce stress and promote relaxation.

Additional Tips

Professional Guidance

It is crucial to consult with healthcare providers, like a primary care physician or physical therapist, before initiating a stretching program for chronic pain. They will assess your condition, recommend appropriate stretches, and ensure your safety.

Pain Assessment

Throughout your stretching routine, closely monitor your body's response. If you experience increased pain or discomfort, consult your healthcare provider to adjust your routine or explore other treatment options.

Gradual Progression

Start your stretching program slowly and progress gradually. Avoid overstretching, which can lead to muscle or joint strain. Gradual progression minimizes the risk of injury.

Consistency

Consistency is key for managing chronic pain through stretching. Incorporate stretching into your daily routine to experience the most significant benefits in pain reduction.

Medication and Other Treatments

Work with your healthcare provider to determine if medications, physical therapy, or complementary treatments (e.g., acupuncture, massage therapy) can enhance the effectiveness of your stretching regimen for pain management.

Stretching for chronic pain management is an integral part of a holistic approach to pain relief. Professional guidance, understanding the type and source of your chronic pain, and selecting the right stretches for your condition are essential for achieving meaningful and sustainable relief.

Contacting a Healthcare Professional

You may be wondering that if you can manage your medical condition by stretching and maintaining a healthy lifestyle, then what's the point of visiting a doctor and following their treatment plan? Here is why. Contacting a healthcare professional is critical when dealing with medical conditions, even if you are incorporating stretching and self-care into your routine. Healthcare professionals play a central role in the management of your condition for several important reasons.

Firstly, they can provide an accurate diagnosis of your medical condition. Many conditions, such as chronic pain or arthritis, have different sub-types, and understanding the specific nature of your condition is essential for effective treatment. Once diagnosed, healthcare providers can create personalized treatment plans that address the unique aspects of your condition. These plans may involve a combination of therapies, medications, lifestyle changes, and exercises, including stretching.

In some cases, medication may be a critical component of your treatment, and healthcare professionals can prescribe and monitor your medications to ensure effectiveness and minimize potential side effects or interactions. They can also refer you to a physical therapist for conditions requiring musculoskeletal rehabilitation. Healthcare providers can monitor your progress through regular check-ups, allowing for the adjustment of your treatment plan as needed. They can order advanced diagnostic tests, such as imaging studies or laboratory tests, to fully understand your condition and provide guidance on safe and effective exercise, including stretching.

Additionally, healthcare professionals offer support and education, helping you understand your condition, its triggers, and how to manage it effectively. This knowledge can empower you to make informed decisions about your health. For complex medical conditions, comprehensive care often involves a team of healthcare professionals, including primary care physicians, specialists, physical therapists, and nurses, working together to manage your condition.

This coordinated approach ensures that you receive the best care possible. While stretching and self-care are valuable components of managing certain medical conditions, they should be part of a broader treatment plan overseen by healthcare professionals. So, consulting your healthcare provider to determine the most suitable approach for your specific medical condition and individual needs is of paramount importance.

Chapter 7: Progression and Challenges

Life is all about progress. If you aren't moving forward, you are standing still, and no one wants that. Naturally, you will want to see real results shortly after you start practicing. Luckily, with stretching, you will notice a difference in the first few weeks, provided you practice regularly. So, what are these changes? Well, this is what you will discover in this chapter.

Similarly, you will also experience challenges. Practicing the same stretches can get boring with time, impacting your body's progress. This happens to everyone. No one likes routine, and even your body needs a challenge and push from time to time. Luckily, there are things you can do to overcome this feeling.

Resistance bands have been mentioned a couple of times in this book, and for good reason. They are necessary in elevating your stretching performance. If you want to progress, you must switch up your routine and add more equipment. This chapter covers various techniques to incorporate resistance bands in your exercises.

How Can You Progress with Stretching?

Generally, you should notice progress after four weeks of stretching. However, some people can practice for months but don't see results. There are things you can do and mistakes you should avoid when achieving your fitness goals.

Don't Train Too Frequently

When you first start stretching, it is normal to feel enthusiastic and want to practice frequently. Some people get excited after learning the many advantages of stretching and believe that constant training will get them fast results. However, this isn't true. The human body, whether old or young, can't tolerate stretching every day. Your body needs a break to repair and revitalize itself after a stretching exercise.

Only train two days a week. You might worry that this won't be enough to achieve real results. However, training every day or more than twice a week can strain your muscles and cause damage. Eventually, you will not be able to continue exercising. So, take it easy and be patient, and you will see progress.

Practice Warm-Up Exercises

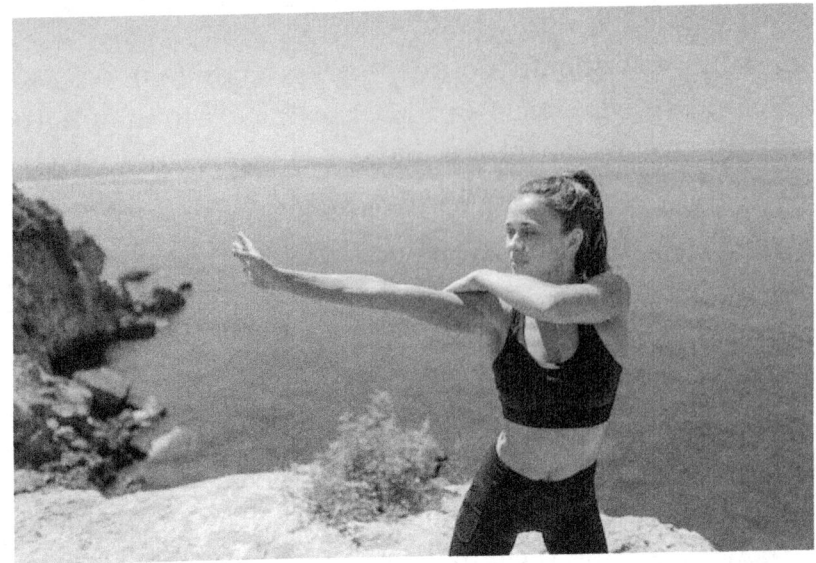

58. These exercises don't only warm up the muscles but also prevent injuries and improve your stretching techniques. Source: https://www.pexels.com/photo/woman-in-black-activewear-stretching-her-arm-8861040/

By now, you understand the significance of warm-up exercises. They are simple movements that can hugely impact your stretching routine, making it more effective. If you perform a gentle stretch or a light exercise, you don't have to warm up every time. However, if you are practicing intense or full-body stretches, like ones that increase flexibility, you should take a few minutes to do warm-up exercises.

These exercises don't only warm up the muscles but also prevent injuries and improve your stretching techniques. If you don't warm up before practicing, you won't get the results you are hoping for, and you will be delaying your progress. It only takes 5 to minutes to do these exercises, but they can make a huge difference.

Don't Push through the Pain

Some people think if they push through the pain when exercising, it will eventually go away. The "No pain, no gain" mentality can make you think that if your body aches, you are doing something right.

However, pain is usually a signal from your body that you should stop and take a break. In this situation, your body is telling you that the stretching exercise is unsafe or you are doing it wrong. If you push through the pain, you can injure your nerves, ligaments, and muscles. It will take months to recover, and you won't be able to exercise, which will affect your progress.

People of all ages can experience pain when stretching, depending on the exercise, their health, and flexibility. Make it a rule to listen to your body and stop right away when you feel something isn't right. Don't let the pain discourage you. There are dozens of stretching techniques in this book, so you will surely find ones that won't be painful.

Stretch with a Proper Form

Having good form while stretching is extremely necessary as it lengthens the targeted muscles without causing stress or tension on the joints or injury. Follow the instructions for every exercise in the book exactly as they are so you can practice with the correct form.

Don't Only Perform Passive Stretches

No one can deny the significance of passive stretches. However, there are several others, and focusing on only one can slow down your progress. Although passive stretches improve mobility, range of motion, and flexibility, they aren't enough by themselves. You need to practice a combination of dynamic, PNF, and other stretches to reap the benefits stretching offers.

Passive stretches are limited. They are ideal for beginners and to prepare your body for more intense stretching exercises. However, if you are seeking progress, you need to switch things up, or you will remain at a beginner level. There are different stretches for a reason. Each has its benefits, so don't deprive yourself of them by focusing on one type.

Focus on Your Goals

Some people workout to lose weight, some to stay fit, while others want to increase their flexibility. Before you start stretching, you should set goals for yourself. What do you hope to achieve? Do you want to improve your mobility, flexibility, balance, etc.? Ask yourself various questions to get an idea of why you want to start this exercise regimen. Once you have the answers, focus on the stretching exercises that will bring you closer to your goals. Many people make the mistake of choosing exercises based on whether they are fun or easy and then wonder why they don't see results.

Choose stretching exercises based on the muscles you want to target. Ask yourself which muscles you want to strengthen or stretch and pick the appropriate exercise. For instance, if you can't bend and reach your toes, focus on exercises that increase your hamstring flexibility.

Understand There Are Different Types of Progress

Progress doesn't look the same for everyone. Some people may see results in a couple of weeks, while for others, it can take months. Two people can practice the same exercise, and each will get a different result. For instance, you and your friend are practicing the same technique for a month. They experience a huge improvement in mobility while you only experience comfort. Both are still considered progress.

Don't compare your progress with anyone else's, and celebrate every goal you achieve, no matter how small. Be patient with yourself and understand that every person progresses at their own pace.

Now that you understand how you can achieve your fitness goals, discover what you will experience when you stretch regularly.

Gradually Increasing Flexibility

As you age, flexibility exercises like stretching become a necessity. Flexibility issues can impact your quality of life and prevent you from doing simple daily tasks, like bending over or stretching your arms to get something off the counter. Regularly practicing stretching can gradually increase flexibility and improve stability.

You will notice progress from two weeks to three months, depending on your age, health conditions, and other factors. However, significant improvements can take six months or longer, but you will only start to see progress when you practice regularly. Since stretching increases blood flow in the body, you will notice an improvement in muscle strength, affecting your posture and mobility. You will move more easily, and exercising will be more fun as you won't exert as much effort as when you first started.

Look at how your body will progress with regular stretching:

Improved Posture

After practicing stretching for a couple of months, you will have a better posture and notice fewer aches.

Increased Stamina

As the blood flows through your body, you will notice an increase in your muscle strength and stamina. You will be able to endure various physical activities without feeling exhausted and fatigued.

Increased Lower Body Flexibility

Practicing ankle stretch and inner thigh stretch exercises will improve lower-body flexibility. You will notice less swelling and strain on your knees and muscles.

Bring Balance and Stability

Stretching increases joint stability and reduces joint pain, which brings awareness to your body. You will notice an improvement in your balance, giving you more independence to do your daily tasks without help.

Reduced Discomfort

Spinal stenosis is a big part of aging that, sadly, no one can avoid and can cause discomfort when performing the simplest tasks. By practicing stretching, you will notice less pain and stress in the joints.

Walking Faster

Lack of flexibility affects your mobility. You walk more slowly, experience back pain, and are prone to falling. Stretching exercises targeting the front hips will substantially impact your walking speed. With regular exercise, you will walk faster, better, and with more stability.

An increase in flexibility relaxes muscles, tendons, and rigid ligaments, resulting in quick movements.

Less Falling and Injuries

Lack of flexibility can affect balance and cause falling and injuries. Regular stretching will increase your flexibility and prevent slips and falls. Since stretching improves your mobility, you will walk with longer steps, reducing the risk of falling.

Other examples of the progress you will notice after a few weeks of training are:

- You will feel stronger, especially when your muscles are strong enough to perform any stretching exercise.

- You won't feel sore after stretching.

- You can perform more complex stretches.

- You will feel comfortable while stretching.

- You will be able to hold the stretch position longer.

Overcoming Plateaus

You won't only experience progression while stretching. You will face some challenges, too. One main issue you could face is the workout plateau. This term describes a stage where your body gets used to the exercise routine, and you stop experiencing progress. Initially, you achieved your goals, but after some time, you notice nothing changing. Even though you are doing everything right, like exercising regularly and performing the right stretch techniques, you have stopped seeing results.

Although workout plateaus happen to everyone, they can be very frustrating. You work hard, eat healthily, and sleep well, but you can't see any progress. For instance, someone exercises to lose weight. At first, everything was going well, and they could see their weight dropping. After a few months, they notice they aren't losing weight even though they work out every day and only eat healthy food. So, where is the problem?

Everyone experiences workout plateaus. It has nothing to do with age, gender, or the exercise they perform. It is just human nature. Any new workout routine is only effective initially. However, if you keep repeating the same exercise over and over for months, your body will get used to it, and the workout will stop being effective. The human body usually adjusts to repeated patterns. In other words, you have done this exercise many times, so your body knows what to expect.

A workout plateau also happens when you exercise every day. If you don't give your muscles time to repair themselves, you will stop seeing progress.

Although plateaus can be very frustrating, they are usually a good sign. Your body is telling you that you have achieved many of your goals, and you should challenge yourself to accomplish more. You can overcome workout plateaus with these simple tips:

Change Your Routine

Regularly switching up your workout routine is one of the most effective ways to overcome a plateau. However, you don't have to change your whole regimen every couple of weeks. Only change the order of the stretches and add a new technique every week or two.

Incorporate new stretches into your routine to target different muscles. Your body is smart, so don't let it get bored, and surprise it with new moves occasionally. Changing your routine keeps you motivated, eliminates boredom, and challenges your body with new exercises so it doesn't get too comfortable.

If you can't come up with new exercises, mixing up the order of the stretches is enough. This simple strategy changes your body's stimulus, which increases its mass and strength. Your body adapts to routine and movements. When you switch up the order of the stretches, you catch it off-guard and keep it guessing.

Also, pay attention to how you respond mentally and physically to every stretch. If an exercise makes you feel burned out or bored, it is time to change your routine. Keep changing things and challenging yourself to overcome plateaus.

Take Breaks

Taking breaks from your exercise routine is essential. You won't only rest your body and mind but will also prevent plateaus. However, you can still be active on your breaks by doing other exercises, like walking, yoga, and swimming. Taking time away from stretching gives you the chance to assess your progress and see if you need to adjust your goals or routine.

Consider More Intense Exercises

What better way to challenge yourself than to increase the intensity of your exercise? You can do this by incorporating resistance bands or dumbbells into your stretching routine. You can also do more repetitions in each stretch to build strength and muscle.

Exercise with a Friend

If you feel unmotivated or stretching has become a tedious task rather than something that refreshes your body and mind, consider working out with a family member or friend. They will challenge you and make exercising fun. You could learn new techniques from each other and push one another to achieve your fitness goals. They can point out when you are exerting too much effort so you can take a break before you hurt yourself.

Choose someone your age that you feel comfortable with to make exercising an enjoyable experience.

Watch What You Eat

You can do everything right and still experience a plateau. If you aren't eating healthily or giving your body the nutrients it needs, it won't give you the results you want. Understand that with age, your body has different nutritional requirements. Focus on eating healthy meals every day. Consult your doctor to determine if there is certain food you should avoid. Make sure to drink enough water every day and never get dehydrated.

Incorporating Resistance Bands

Resistance bands should be incorporated into your exercise routine. If you want to advance in your workout routine and achieve more goals, start exercising with these bands.

Here are some simple resistance band workouts:

Chest Pull

Instructions:

1. Sit up straight on a comfortable chair with your feet on the ground and slightly apart.

2. Hold the resistance band at both ends and bring it in front of your chest.

3. Breathe out while pulling the band and straightening your arms to the front. Where? To the front? Sides?

4. Breathe in, then release the band.

5. Repeat 10 times.

The Bent Over Technique

Instructions:

1. Sit on a chair with your feet on the floor slightly apart.

2. Hold both ends of the resistance band tight with both hands and stand on your resistance band with your feet.

3. Bend your body forward, pull the resistance band's handles with your hands upward, and take a deep breath. Your elbows should be facing the ceilings.

4. Breathe out, then release the band.

5. Repeat 10 times or more if you can.

Lateral Raise

Instructions:

1. Stand in the middle of your resistance band with both feet flat on the ground.

2. With your arms at your sides, hold the band's handles

3. Raise your arms to the side at the height of your shoulders, then lower them again.

4. Repeat 10 times.

Five Squats

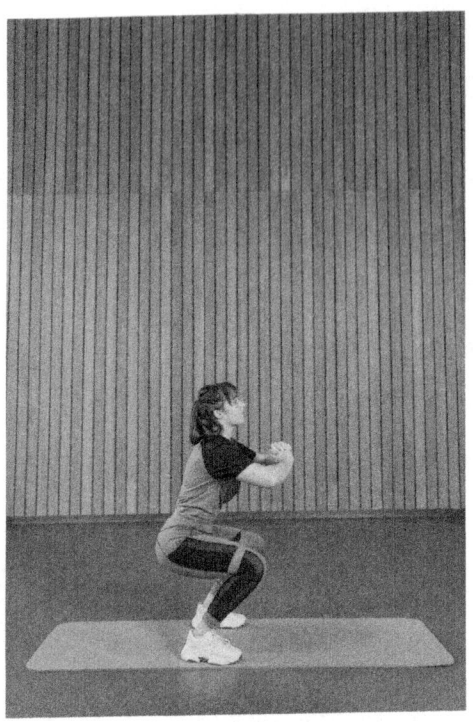

59. Bend your knees as if you are squatting with your butt out and your back straightened. Source: https://www.pexels.com/photo/a-woman-standing-on-a-mat-doing-the-squats-with-a-resistance-band-6339648/

Instructions:

1. Stand in the middle of your resistance band with both arms by your sides and hold it on both ends.

2. Bend your knees as if you are squatting with your butt out and your back straightened.

3. Repeat 10 times.

Chest Press

Instructions:

1. Sit down or stand. Choose what makes you comfortable with both feet together on the floor.

2. Hold the resistance band on both ends, then place it behind your shoulders.

3. Extend your arms forward and bring them to your chest, then release.

4. Repeat 10 times.

Leg Press

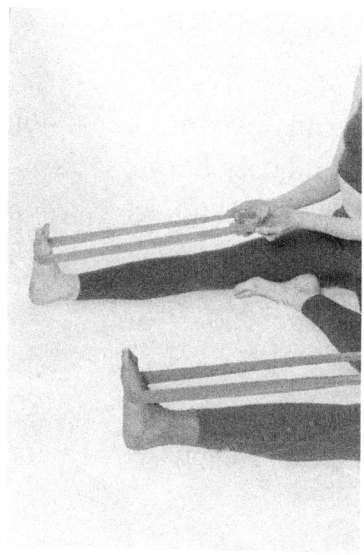

60. Slightly lift your left foot, then place it in the middle of the band.
Source: https://www.pexels.com/photo/crop-athletes-stretching-resistance-loops-during-training-7479763/

Instructions:

1. Sit up straight on a chair with your back straight and feet together on the floor.

2. Grip the resistance band on both ends.

3. Slightly lift your left foot, then place it in the middle of the band. Your left foot and band should be off the ground, while your right foot should be on the floor. Keep your back straight.

4. Bend your left knee toward you, then straighten it.

5. Then, return to the first position.

6. Repeat the previous steps with your right foot.

7. Repeat the exercise 10 times with each foot.

Triceps Press

Instructions:

1. Stand and put your left heel under one end of the resistance band.

2. With both hands by your sides, hold the other end of the stretch band with both hands.

3. Stretch upward over your head, then release.

4. Repeat 10 times.

Calf Press

Instructions:

1. Sit up straight on a chair with feet together on the ground.

2. Slightly lift your left foot and place the resistance band under it.

3. Hold the band on both ends with both hands.

4. Extend your left leg straight out in front with your toes pointing upward.

5. Next, flex and point your toes downward.

6. Repeat the previous steps with your right leg.

7. Repeat 10 times.

Resistance Bands Challenges

You might face a few challenges when you start using resistance bands. Luckily, for every problem, there is a solution.

- Your hands may hurt from holding the band or adding pressure to it while exercising. To solve this problem, choose a padded band that feels comfortable in your hands.

- It can feel uncomfortable or strange when using a resistance band for the first time. This is normal; with constant practice, you will get used to it.

Whatever you do in life, you will always face challenges. Experiencing a workout plateau can be frustrating. You keep working hard, and you don't see results. However, you shouldn't give up. Plateaus indicate you have achieved some of your goals, and you need to make adjustments to keep progressing. Changing your routine and challenging your body can prevent boredom and keep you motivated.

Pay attention to your body, and you will notice progress. Any positive change should be welcomed and recognized as a step toward achieving your goals. Keep working on yourself and follow the tips in this book, and you will see a change in a matter of weeks. However, understand that achieving your goals takes time, and everyone progresses at their own pace. Be patient with yourself if it takes you longer, and believe you will eventually get where you want to be.

Chapter 8: Staying Safe

Despite its many benefits, stretching still has its risks. Learning how to perform the exercises safely is the best way to start your journey to improved mobility and flexibility. As a senior, you must be mindful of the risks associated with physical exercise.

This chapter outlines the pivotal safety guidelines and precautions recommended when doing stretching workouts. It talks about the most common stretching mistakes and how to avoid them and provides tips and tricks for preventing injuries or strains effectively. Last but not least, this chapter emphasizes the importance of consulting with your healthcare provider before starting a new workout, including stretching. Besides giving additional advice on how to tailor exercises to prevent mishaps, your doctor can help you determine which exercises are safe and explain how your health condition affects your ability to work out. Whether familiarizing yourself with stretching or an experienced practitioner, these safety guidelines and precautions will help you maximize your workout's benefits while minimizing the risk of injury.

Common Stretching Mistakes

Maintaining proper form is essential when performing stretching exercises to prevent injury and make the most of your workout. Carefully follow the instructions for each movement and position, and engage the proper muscles to keep your body in the correct posture. Besides this, there are several other ways to avoid common stretching mistakes. Below are some errors beginners often make and tips on how to sidestep them.

Rushing through the Workout

When movement is required between the positions, novice practitioners try to switch too quickly, making sudden movements. Besides this resulting in most cases, it also represents a greater risk of injury, especially for seniors. By keeping your motions controlled and smooth, you'll ensure your muscles are working effectively, help you maintain proper form and alignment, and avoid injuries and strains.

Trying to Work through the Pain

While you might experience a little discomfort when you start stretching, you shouldn't feel pain. If you do, it's a sign you aren't doing the exercise properly or have pushed your body too hard. Experiencing pain during the entire workout is normal for some people if they haven't exercised in a while. However, by fighting to work through pain, you're minimizing the stretching benefits and ignoring a strain or injury. Remember to listen to your body. If you experience pain or discomfort, stop the exercise immediately and make necessary adjustments to your form.

Skipping Warm-Up Exercises

Since it's a low-intensity workout, many think of stretching as warming up. However, by not warming up your muscles before stretching, you're making it harder for them to work during the exercise. By contrast, a 5-minute pre-stretch warm-up is ideal for boosting blood flow through your body, allowing it to perform different movements. Whether walking or just moving your limbs, warming up should be a cardinal part of every exercise.

Doing Improper Stretching Techniques

Most people associate stretching with static stretching, which is holding a position for a few seconds until you feel the tension in the affected muscle group. This is recommended as a post-workout or during any workout exercise. Doing this at the beginning of your workout isn't ideal because it increases the risk of injuries. On the other hand, dynamic stretching is moving slowly, which is fantastic for warming up the muscles and joints. Mastering the proper exercise techniques and following the steps are essential to achieve the best results. It includes using the correct posture, executing a complete range of motion, and incorporating breathing techniques to optimize the workouts for each stretching exercise.

Bouncing While Stretching

Even if you're doing dynamic stretching, you should never bounce with your entire body. Otherwise, you'll end up with pulled muscles and aching joints and will be unable to stretch for a while. Muscle pulling happens when a sudden motion (like bouncing) causes the muscle tissues to tighten to shield themselves from tearing. Instead of bouncy movements, work on gradually lengthening the time it takes for you to do a dynamic stretch exercise.

Not Stretching Often Enough

Your workouts should be tailored to your needs and capabilities, but exercising as frequently as possible is pivotal. If you start skipping sessions, you might risk getting injured because your muscles have to relearn the movements and get used to relaxing and lengthening excessively again. Moreover, if you aren't stretching often enough, you won't see many benefits from your workout. By contrast, you can improve or maintain your muscle and joint flexibility and improve your quality of life with regular stretching workouts.

Not Stretching for Long Enough

When doing static stretches, many fall into the mistake of not holding a pose long enough. While initially, you might think holding a particularly challenging pose for the predetermined time is unnecessary or impossible, it's crucial not to give up unless you feel extreme pain, dizziness, or other intense discomfort. Holding a stretch long enough enables your muscles to relax and release their tightness.

Holding Your Breath

Unintentionally holding their breath is another common mistake people make while stretching. This mistake partially stems from trying too hard to do the exercise right, so they take a deep breath and forget to release it before moving into the stretching position. By doing so, they deprive their muscles of oxygen, which causes them to tense and resist stretching. However, by continuing to breathe through the nose while holding a pose, your muscles can relax and extend.

Stretching Injured Muscles

When you injure a muscle, you're tearing the muscle tissue, which needs time to heal. Strengthening it will exacerbate the condition and prolong the time your body requires to restore the injured tissue to its healthy state. So, if you injure a muscle during stretching, do your best to rest it and wait until it heals before you start working it again with low-intensity exercises.

Not Wearing Proper Shoes and Clothing

Another mistake people make when performing a low-intensity exercise like stretching is thinking any clothes and shoes will do for the workout. However, by wearing ill-fitting clothing, you're risking injury. Tight clothes limit your movements, which might cause your muscles to tighten and get strained. To optimize your stretching workouts, always wear loose-fitting, comfy clothes, allowing a free range of movement for all muscle groups. Likewise, wear properly fitting shoes suitable for this activity. Investing in a pair with proper arch support and cushioned heels for added shock absorption is a good idea. These will be useful in exercises where you have to shift balance.

Not Starting with the Appropriate Intensity

Assessing current fitness levels is pivotal before you start performing any exercise. Knowing your physical fitness levels makes it easier to determine which movements and routines will work best for improving your muscle strength, which is essential for stretching. At the same time, by evaluating your body's strength, balance, flexibility, endurance, and overall health, you'll identify your limitations.

If you're new to stretching, the worst thing you can do is to jump right in starting intermediate or high-level exercises. Despite being a low-impact workout, stretching can quickly lead to serious injuries if you start working with stiff muscles and joints that aren't used to relaxing and elongating regularly. Start slowly with beginner-friendly movements and only move up levels when you become comfortable doing these.

Stretching When You're Ill

Even if you have a common cold or flu, stretching can further drain your body of the energy it desperately needs to heal itself. Moreover, suppose you attempt to exercise when feeling unwell. In that case, you cannot focus on maintaining the proper form and balance. Take time off and allow your body to heal for at least a week (depending on your illness) to avoid injuries and prolong your recovery.

Not Listening to Your Body Afterward

Even if you don't feel pain but your joints and muscles feel tight or sore days after stretching, it's a sign you've put too much strain on them during your workout. It indicates that you should try a lower-intensity session instead to give your body a chance to adapt to the movements and the pressure. Don't try to soldier through the discomfort, especially if you experience this every time you do a stretching workout. It's unnecessary and won't get you closer to your flexibility goal. In most cases, it will do more harm than good, especially for seniors.

Injury Prevention Tips

The most common injuries associated with stretching are the consequences of overuse. Repeating the same movement or exercise repeatedly without rest or with improper form leads to muscle strain, inflammation, and pain. It happens when you focus too much on one part of your body, neglecting other areas, or do too much too soon without allowing your body time to adjust. To prevent injuries and strain caused by overuse, start slowly and gradually increase your workouts' intensity and duration. In addition, take appropriate breaks and modify exercises as needed. If you experience pain or discomfort during your session, stop immediately and consult your healthcare provider, who can help determine whether you've injured yourself or have a preexisting condition needing treatment.

Maintaining proper form is the first tenet of avoiding injury during this type of workout. However, it's even more critical to maintain good form and use the appropriate technique to avoid injury if you're using additional equipment. Here are a few examples of preexisting conditions that might limit your ability to do certain stretching exercises:

- **Arthritis:** If you have arthritis issues, you should avoid stretching exercises that put too much strain on your joints, whether by overloading them with your body weight or stretching the same body parts for a long period. Instead, prioritize exercises that improve joint mobility and flexibility.

- **Back Pain:** If you suffer from back pain, you should avoid exercises that exacerbate your pain and further strain your back muscles. The exercises to avoid are those that stretch your back and core muscles and require you to hold a pose using these muscle groups almost exclusively. Instead, focus on exercises that improve your posture and promote a pain-free back.

- **Diabetes:** If you have diabetes, avoid exercises that cause a sudden drop in blood sugar levels. These include activities with sudden movements and those requiring your legs to be higher than your head and vital organs, as they disrupt normal blood circulation through the body and cause blood stagnation in certain body parts. Instead, focus on exercises that promote blood flow and balance blood sugar levels and require slow, deliberate movements.

- **High Blood Pressure:** If you have high blood pressure, avoiding movements requiring you to hold your breath or strain your neck is crucial. These movements put pressure on your lungs and airways, causing them to struggle to provide enough oxygen to your body, which further raises blood pressure. Instead, opt for poses that'll keep your blood pressure levels steady.

- **Injured Spinal Discs**: If you have a herniated disc, stay away from poses involving bending or twisting your spine. Instead, focus on exercises that strengthen your core muscles so you can use these to improve your posture instead of relying on your spine to support your balance during the session.

- **Joint Replacement:** If you have undergone joint replacement surgery, it's best to avoid poses that will put excessive strain on your new joint and surrounding tissue. Instead, focus on movements promoting joint mobility and stability to foster a faster healing process and help you regain the joint's mobility.

- **Multiple Sclerosis (MS):** Avoid exercises that cause muscle fatigue or exacerbate neurological symptoms if you have MS. They include stretches that require quick repositioning and holding long positions and anything that strains the spine. Instead, opt for exercises to improve muscle strength and stability.

- **Osteoporosis:** If you have osteoporosis, exercises that strain your spine or involve twisting movements might aggravate your condition. Leave these out of your repertoire and focus on positions that build bone density instead.

- **Pulmonary Diseases:** If you have asthma, emphysema, bronchitis, COPD, or other chronic pulmonary conditions, avoid movements that cause shortness of breath or excessive exertion. These include stretching exercises, causing you to breathe faster and harder. Focusing on poses that improve lung function and teach you how to breathe properly is more beneficial for avoiding complications and further aggravating your condition.

Another way to prevent injuries is to focus not only on warming up but on cooling down, too. Your muscles and joints need a little time to cool down after your workout, so aim to move your body a little more slowly than usual. If you're working out in warmer conditions, you need more time to cool down but less to warm up. Whereas if you're stretching in colder conditions, you need longer to warm up your muscles and joints and less to cool them down. However, avoid cooling down too quickly, as this could be detrimental to your joints.

By avoiding some exercises and focusing on those that are safe for your body, you can enjoy the benefits of stretching without risking injury. However, remember everyone's body is different, and what is safe for one person might not be safe for another. If you have a preexisting medical condition, this is all the more reason to consult a healthcare provider before beginning an exercise program.

Consultation with a Healthcare Professional

As eager and motivated as you might be to start a new exercise routine as a senior, consulting your healthcare provider before you embark on this journey is essential. Whether you have preexisting conditions or not, preserving your health is of utmost importance. Hence, having reassurance that the workout you've chosen (in this case, stretching) is safe for you is imperative.

Your body changes as you age, and what you could do easily when you were younger might not be a suitable option anymore. Consult a healthcare provider before starting your stretching workout. This can help you avoid potential injuries and set reasonable and achievable goals. Your physician will recommend modifications or alternative exercises that suit your age and fitness level.

If you're considering adding stretching to your daily schedule, make an appointment with your doctor (primary or specialist, depending on whether you have a preexisting condition). Prepare a list of questions to ask your doctor to get the most information during your consultation and safely start your exercises. Here are a few suggestions:

- What stretching exercises would work best based on your current activity level and condition?

- Are there specific movements or poses you should avoid based on your medical history and current conditions? For example, if you have a hernia, ask if it's okay to stretch the affected muscle group based on its current level of healing.

- Is there anything you should do or avoid if you're preparing for surgery or worried about getting blood clots?

- Bring up unexplained symptoms if you've been experiencing any. For example, if you felt joint pain, chest pain, shortness of breath (with or without light exercise like walking up the stairs), dizziness, sores that won't heal, or swelling unrelated to a diagnosed condition. Ask the doctor if it's a good idea to start exercising despite these or if you should postpone your workout.

- How does your health condition affect your ability to exercise? If you have a chronic or acute health condition, discuss this thoroughly with the appropriate healthcare provider. Ask them whether they can recommend adjustments to tailor your stretching workout to your needs and abilities so you can get the most out of them without risking injuries.

- Ask whether preventive care is up to date. You might need to do further testing before you can start exercising, especially if you haven't done any lately. Even if you're feeling well, stretching will put added strain on your body and bring out hidden injury or illness. For example, women over 60 are at a higher risk of osteoporosis (and consequently bone breaks) than men of the same age and should be checked more frequently.

Start with the Proper Plan

Another reason to consult a healthcare provider before beginning an exercise program is they can help you devise a plan to gradually and safely increase the duration and intensity of your physical activity. Look at it as a prescription, like part of a conventional treatment. After all, stretching is a form of self-healing as it improves your mobility and fitness and helps prevent and alleviate numerous conditions.

As part of your prescription, the doctor can help you formulate short-term and long-term fitness goals. Setting goals will give you a sense of direction. For example, if you can only hold a certain pose for a short period, your short-term goal could be to work on maintaining it longer. Long-term goals could be alleviating back pain or similar symptoms. Setting similar goals also keeps you motivated as you'll be working toward crucial milestones you set for yourself. By improving your flexibility and mobility, you gain a sense of accomplishment, keeping you motivated in the long run. Moreover, tracking progress becomes easier when you have a goal to follow. By seeing the improvements you've made, you can adjust the routine accordingly.

As with other prescriptions, when you go for refills, your doctor can help you review your treatment plan and see whether you are on the right path toward your long-term goals. Personalizing goals becomes easier as you can focus more on the areas that need improvements, like adding exercises to improve strength and balance or relieving painful conditions.

They can help you tailor and adjust your goals as you progress in building your stretching abilities or if something comes up and you must take a rest. It doesn't necessarily have to be an illness. You might go on a vacation where you want to take a break from exercising. If you take a longer break and have a preexisting condition, consulting your doctor again before you start stretching anew is a good idea.

While stretching is a great way to improve your mobility and flexibility, your workout program should be tailor-made for you. It should be suitable for your specific needs and health conditions. By consulting your physician, you gain guidance on how to modify each exercise to suit your current abilities and reduce the risk of injury. You might be advised to avoid certain activities right away. However, this doesn't have to mean you won't be able to do them in the future. You might need to leave them out of your regime for a while and revisit them when you've recovered, or you might work on gradually incorporating them into your routine with the proper guidance of an experienced professional.

By consulting your doctor before starting to incorporate stretching workouts into your routine, you ensure that you're taking the right steps to preserve your health while minimizing the risk of injury. So, make an appointment with your healthcare provider and discuss your plans to start your new exercise plans. Based on your unique needs and medical history, they can advise you on the best steps for moving forward with your exercise regime.

Chapter 9: Lifestyle and Well-Being

While inherently beneficial, like many other forms of physical exercise, stretching alone won't be enough to make you fit and healthy. You also have to implement other lifestyle changes to improve your well-being and maximize your workout's benefits. These lifestyle changes encompass the decisions you make regarding your diet, sleep, and other habits.

This chapter provides guidance and advice on how to build and maintain a healthy lifestyle alongside your stretching workouts to help you get started on the journey of transforming your life. You'll learn how seniors can buttress their flexibility through nutrition, the role hydration plays in stretching benefits, and how stress reduction contributes to your wellness.

Nutrition for Flexibility

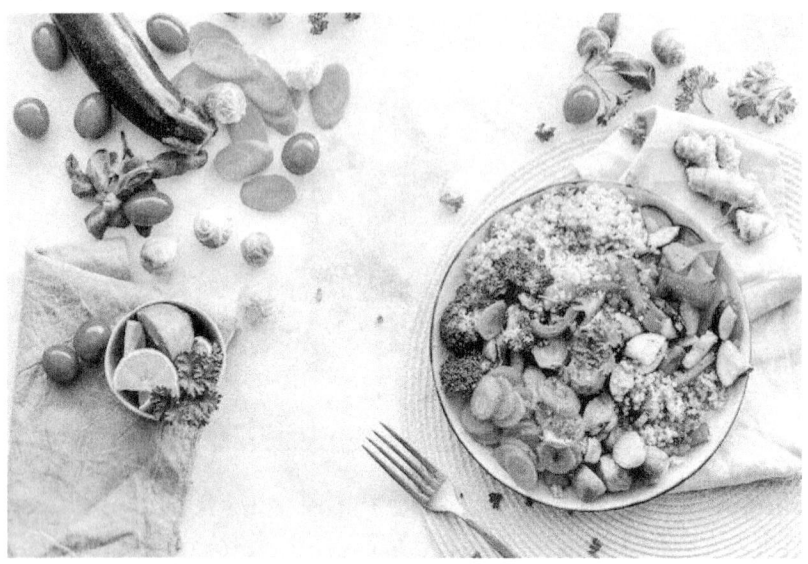

61. Since your body changes with age, so do your nutritional needs. Source: https://www.pexels.com/photo/flat-lay-photography-of-vegetable-salad-on-plate-1640777/

Unhealthy diets can cause health conditions like cardiovascular issues, diabetes, high cholesterol, tooth decay, high blood pressure, obesity, and cancer, all of which are more prevalent in seniors. Since your body changes with age, so do your nutritional needs. Understanding what your body needs to remain healthy and active is crucial for establishing a balanced diet. A healthy diet will protect you against various diseases, keep you fit, and provide more energy for your workouts and daily tasks. However, besides gaining all these benefits, you can use your diet to gain more flexibility, making your stretching workouts more effective. Below are a few tips on what to incorporate into your diet.

Foods for Improving Circulation

The best foods for improving circulation contain omega-3 fatty acids, like fish, flax and pumpkin seeds, nuts, and olive oil. These help keep the blood vessels clean and flexible, allowing blood to flow uninterrupted. Foods rich in anti-inflammatory agents (like green vegetables and fruit) have a similar effect.

Food to Boost Your Energy

Older adults often struggle with workouts due to a lack of energy. One of the causes behind this might be anemia, a condition that can be remedied by eating food rich in iron, like red meat, spinach, or eggs. Avoid refined carbohydrates like sugary food, white bread, pizza, white flour, pasta, and white rice, as these cause sudden sugar spikes and drops (you'll have even less energy once the sugar is metabolized). Opt for complex carbs instead, like vegetables and whole grains, to boost your energy, as these are high in fiber and low in calories.

Food for Bone Health

Your diet should contain plenty of vitamin D and calcium to prevent bone loss. Besides natural sunlight, the best sources of vitamin D are eggs, dairy, mushrooms, and salmon. Leafy green vegetables, oatmeal, and dried fruit like figs and raisins are packed with calcium.

Anti-Inflammatory Foods

Food high in saturated fat and processed sugar leads to inflammation in the body, often causing bloating and muscle and joint stiffness. As these foods aren't meant to be used by the body, it doesn't know what to do with them and reacts with inflammation. To avoid inflammation getting in your way of improving your flexibility, stay clear of unhealthy foods and opt for nutrient-dense, anti-inflammatory produce instead. Some examples are nuts (Brazil, macadamia, walnuts, almonds, and cashews), green leafy vegetables (collards, arugula, kale, and spinach), fish, berries, and other fresh fruit like oranges and cherries, and spices (including turmeric, ginger, chili peppers, and cinnamon).

Besides being a fantastic tool for reducing inflammation-induced symptoms, consuming anti-inflammatory foods also does wonders for improving your mental health. Without stiffness, pain, or bloating limiting you, you'll be much more motivated to work out. You'll have the willpower and mental energy to focus on performing your stretching exercises, and you will soon see the benefits of your hard work.

Foods Supportive Connective Tissue Health

To boost your flexibility through nutrition, paying attention to your connective tissue's health is advisable. Consisting of tendons, fascia, and ligaments, connective tissue supports your muscles and bones, making it indispensable for building and maintaining a healthy, flexible body. To properly nurture your connective tissues, you must up your collagen intake because, as your body ages, it will make less of this essential nutrient. The best natural source of collagen is bone broth.

Berries, broccoli, kiwis, and foods high in vitamin C foster natural collagen production in the body and the production of connective tissue components. However, vitamin C is an unstable vitamin and degrades in heat. It's best to eat food containing this vitamin raw or after as little cooking as possible.

You don't have to start buying and eating all these foods right away. After all, changing a well-established diet (as unhealthy as it may be) takes time. However, you can start slowly incorporating changes in small steps. For example, swap white bread or pasta for a whole-grain version one or two days a week. Making your plate colorful is another way to add more variety to your diet. Vegetables like peppers, tomatoes, or radishes are high in nutrients, delicious, and will make the dish look inviting. Herbs and spices like rosemary, sage, basil, or pepper will add flavor to your meals and make them easier to digest, reducing inflammation. Consider swapping your snacks for healthy options like fruit and vegetable sticks.

Plan your meals and reduce temptation. It might be more convenient to reach for prepackaged food choices, but they're unhealthy and won't do you any good in terms of improving your flexibility and mobility. Planning your meals gives you time to choose and prepare healthy food. At the end of each week, make a list of what you want to eat for the next week and buy all the ingredients. Alternatively, prepare larger batches of healthy meals and store them in the freezer. Or, if you can't cook them, and if your budget allows, order healthy food. Nowadays, food delivery services are not limited to unhealthy fast food anymore. You can choose from numerous healthy options, and when you find what fits your dietary needs, you can get nutritious home-cooked meals delivered to your doorstep. Remove unhealthy food from your home to avoid giving in to temptation.

Last but not least, if you have a serious deficiency in nutrients essential for flexibility and mobility, consider supplements. But consult your healthcare providers first to determine which supplements you need. For example, your doctor might prescribe vitamin D and calcium supplements to support your diet.

Hydration and Stretching

Just as you need a balanced diet to stay healthy and optimize your stretching workouts, you should also pay attention to your hydration. Dehydration can make you feel tired because it lowers your energy and impairs brain, kidney, and digestive tract function. Here are a few more reasons to stay hydrated.

You Won't Notice You Are Dehydrated

When a person starts to feel thirsty, they've already lost 2% of their body fluids, and dehydration has already begun. As people get older, their ability to feel thirst and retain water in the body decreases. Not paying attention to whether you're thirsty and losing water puts you at a greater risk of serious diseases. Certain medications, diabetes, and conditions that cause excessive sweating and diarrhea, and those who lose large quantities of blood are even more exposed to dehydration.

Your Kidney Function Decreases

Your kidneys, the organs responsible for removing unwanted waste by filtering your blood and making urine, control your body's fluid levels. Their function decreases with age, causing them to struggle with waste removal because they can't produce enough urine (or can't do it fast enough). Furthermore, if you don't drink enough liquids, you're putting even more strain on your kidneys and causing even more unfiltered waste to accumulate in your body.

Urinary Incontinence Leads to Further Dehydration

Besides being uncomfortable and more likely to occur during workouts, urinary incontinence also leads to further fluid loss. Those with this condition often avoid drinking water to prevent mishaps when exercising, putting themselves at a greater risk of health conditions. The most common complication is UTIs (urinary tract infections). These happen because the urine naturally contains certain bacteria, but when it's retained, the number of bacteria rises, causing an infection. UTIs are painful and can also cause cognitive symptoms like confusion.

Dehydration Affects Cognitive Functions

Dehydration can leave you confused and impair your ability to learn, remember, and think critically. The reason is that the blood's function to supply nutrients to your organs is compromised. When you don't drink enough water, your blood becomes thicker and unable to carry as many nutrients, leaving your organs to starve. Your brain is one of the largest nutrient consumers in the body. Hence, it's among the first to suffer.

Slower Digestion

Digestion also slows with age, which, combined with an unhealthy diet, often leads to constipation. Not drinking enough liquids further raises this risk and other gastrointestinal symptoms and conditions like acid reflux, gastritis, and ulcers. When you're dehydrated, your stomach either produces digestive acids at the wrong time (when you're not eating and digesting food) or does not produce them at all.

Hydration Aids Your Workouts

Drinking enough fluids helps regulate your body temperature so you can warm up and cool down adequately when you exercise. Moreover, without enough fluids in your body, your joints can't lubricate themselves, making your workouts very painful.

Dehydration Leads to Low Blood Pressure

By decreasing blood volume, dehydration also lowers blood pressure to dangerous levels. As a result, you might feel faint and unable to focus on different tasks and exercises. You'll struggle with maintaining balance and risk falling during your stretching exercises.

For these reasons, seniors are advised to pay attention to drinking enough water to prevent dehydration. Below are tips on how to improve your water intake to stay healthy and fit.

Drink More Water

This is the obvious first step, yet it is where many people fail because they don't remember to drink enough. An average person needs at least 8 glasses of water a day, and if they are active, they need even more. Seniors might also need additional hydration, so aim to have around 9 glasses a day. However, consult your doctor first if you're unsure how much you should drink because certain conditions (like heart disease) might limit the amount of water you can drink.

Set reminders on your phone or alarm clock or place visual reminders near sinks to remember to drink regularly throughout the day. You can also incorporate drinking water into your routines. For example, drinking a glass could be the first step of your morning routine, or you can drink one with every meal. As soon as something becomes a routine, you won't forget to do it.

Consume Foods with High Water Content

Fresh fruits and vegetables like oranges, grapes, watermelon, cucumbers, and tomatoes are naturally made mostly of water. Incorporating them into your meals and snacks will help you stay hydrated.

Be Mindful of Your Activities

Activities like stretching increases the risk of dehydration. If you're exercising outside on a hot summer day, you'll sweat more, and your fluid intake will increase. Drink plenty of water before and after your workouts.

Carry a Water Bottle with You

As an alternative, carry a water bottle with you so you can drink on the go. Investing in an insulator bottle is a phenomenal idea, especially if you like your water chilled. You'll have constant access to water and zero excuses not to drink it. Or, if you find drinking plain water all the time boring, consider alternatives like infusing water with fruit or drinking broths and soups. You can carry these with you, too, and use them to boost your fluid intake.

Be Careful with Other Drinks

Alcohol and caffeinated beverages increase the risk of dehydration because they draw water away from your cells. Have you ever noticed feeling thirsty or having an extremely dry mouth after drinking 1-2 glasses of wine? This is a sign of dehydration. Those who have a lower tolerance for alcohol are at an even greater risk. Besides limiting your alcohol intake, you should swap your coffee for tea (black and green tea blends are a great alternative).

Stress Reduction Techniques

Stress can cause numerous physical and mental health conditions and decrease your energy and motivation for working out. Stress reduction techniques like meditation, visualization, and breathing exercises slow your heart rate and lower your blood pressure, effectively relaxing your mind and body.

Breathing Exercise

Breathing exercises are useful when stressed or overwhelmed.

Instructions:

1. Sit in a comfortable position or lie down.

2. Close your eyes or keep them open, depending on what feels comfortable.

3. Slightly open your mouth and press your tongue on your mouth's roof.

4. Exhale, pushing all the air out of your lungs.

5. Close your mouth, take a deep breath through your nose, and count to 8. If you can't hold your breath this long, count to 4.

6. Slowly breathe out while counting to 8 (or 4).

7. Repeat steps 4-6 steps 4 times.

Meditation

Incorporate this technique into your daily routine by taking a few minutes to meditate at a convenient time. For example, you might find it easier to relax in the morning when everything is still peaceful and quiet. Others might opt for evening sessions for better sleep.

Instructions:

1. Find a quiet room with no distractions.

2. Sit in a comfortable position on a chair, mat, or pillow.

3. Make sure your posture is correct, and straighten your back if you notice you're beginning to slouch.

4. Close your eyes, relax your facial muscles, and slightly open your mouth.

5. Take slow, deep breaths to relax your body.

6. Clear your mind and focus on what you feel and think in the present moment.

7. Stressful or negative thoughts will likely creep into your mind. While they might be distressing, try not to suppress them. Instead, remain calm, acknowledge these thoughts, and keep focusing on your breathing until they pass.

8. Stay with your thoughts for 15 minutes until you feel serene and relaxed.

Visualization

Like meditation, visualization also requires a bit more focus and effort to let go of stressful and negative thoughts and quiet your mind.

Instructions:

1. Sit in a quiet room, make yourself comfortable, and close your eyes.

2. Breathe in and out slowly and deeply to focus your attention and calm yourself down.

3. Visualize yourself in a beautiful place where you feel happy and comfortable.

4. Imagine yourself laughing, relaxed, and feeling happy.

5. Focus on everything around you, notice every detail, and engage all of your senses. Listen to the sound

around you, smell the air, feel its temperature, and take in the sights in front of you.

6. Remain in this place for 10 minutes or until you feel completely serene.

7. When you're ready, return to the present moment and slowly open your eyes.

Journaling

Keeping a journal is another way to become more mindful of distressing thoughts, enabling you to deal with them healthily.

Instructions:

1. When you're getting ready to go to bed, go through the experiences you had during the day and write them down. Your mind will do this naturally, so you'll only have to follow its clues.

2. Relax and focus on stressful situations. Try to remember events when you've found yourself becoming anxious.

3. Go through your notes at the end of each week and again at the end of the month. Notice patterns appearing in your thoughts, feelings, and behaviors.

4. By uncovering these issues, you're enabling yourself to deal with them instead of keeping them hidden in the back of your mind.

Learning to be Present

This mindfulness technique is based on a meditative practice, allowing you to be alone with your thoughts.

Instructions:

1. Start by getting into a comfortable position.

2. Keep your breath regular and let it anchor you as you are doing the exercise.

3. Close your eyes and focus on the natural sensations you experience in your body and mind. Notice any thoughts, feelings, sounds, images, smells, or anything else you perceive.

4. Be aware of what you feel, but don't investigate where the sensations come from.

5. Hone in on your thoughts and feelings and be mindful of them.

6. Now, let go of everything with a large exhale.

Getting Enough Sleep

One reason you might struggle to do your stretching exercises is a lack of sleep, which, in turn, might be caused by stress. Getting a good night's sleep has proven beneficial for a person's physical and mental health. REM sleep is particularly vital for enabling the mind to process information while taking a break, whereas deep sleep allows the body to repair itself. However, your sleep pattern changes with age because your REM and deep sleep stages become shorter. Some seniors struggle with falling asleep, while others wake up multiple times during the night.

Building sleep-friendly routines can help reduce stress and other symptoms causing sleep deprivation. If you haven't got one already, start by getting a comfortable mattress that won't leave you tossing and turning during the night. This is a guaranteed way to avoid waking up stressed in the morning.

You'll know it's time to change your mattress if you keep waking up with a stiff neck or back in the mornings.

Keep a regular sleeping schedule by waking up and going to bed at the same time every day. It sets your body's internal clock and maintains its timing so you can sleep better at night and wake up rested the next morning. Even when you don't get enough sleep, you should still wake up at the same time each day to avoid messing up your new routine.

If you want to relax by reading or listening to music, do it in another room as your bedroom should only be used for sleeping. This will train your body and mind into thinking that once you're in the bedroom, it is time to fall asleep. Exercising at night time might also help you fall asleep faster. However, if possible, don't do this in the bedroom either. You should avoid working out too close to your bedtime as it could make it harder to fall asleep, making you frustrated.

It's also a good idea to avoid stimulants like caffeine 8 hours before going to sleep. Caffeine takes 12 hours to be eliminated from your system. Even in small amounts (like the amounts left after 6 hours), caffeine can keep you up all night. Gadgets are also stimulants, so keep your cell phone, tablet, laptop, and TV out of your bedroom. These devices release blue light that tricks your brain into thinking it's not time to go to bed yet. Moreover, stimulants also increase stress because they're addictive. The more you use them, the more you crave them, and when you don't use them for a long time, you get anxious.

Develop a routine including the same activities each night about an hour before sleep to enable your body to prepare for bed. For example, listen to calming music, read, or take a warm bath to relax. While there's nothing wrong with taking a few minutes to relax, long naps will make it hard to fall asleep at night. Keep yourself occupied during the day so you can stay awake. If you must sleep during the day, take a short nap for about twenty minutes to boost your energy. Do this in the early afternoon to prepare your body and mind to sleep in the evening.

Make your bedroom comfortable, dark, and quiet so you can fall asleep quickly each night. Turn your lights off, shut the blinds, buy cozy covers and blankets, and make sure the room's temperature is ideal for sleep (it should be slightly cooler than usual).

Chapter 10: Success Stories

This final chapter provides testimonials and motivations not only for seniors but also for others who struggle with life-altering joint and muscle conditions. All of the people whose stories are told in this chapter didn't think it possible to recover and achieve a better quality of life. They embarked on truly inspiring stretching and fitness journeys expecting, at best, some relief. Reading this chapter, you'll come across firsthand testimonials from people who changed their lives and achieved extraordinary feats through stretching exercises.

Tina's Hip Pain Management

Tina had suffered from excruciating hip pain for years, and all the doctors she visited told her she would eventually have to undergo hip replacement surgery. However, until then, she needed something, aside from drugs, to alleviate her pain. Tina's daughter insisted she try stretching exercises, particularly Fascial Stretch Therapy, which targets the fascia and joints, for pain management. Although she was reluctant at first, Tina was in desperate need of relief and decided to try it. She didn't know that from that moment on, her life would change forever.

Nellie's Health and Lifestyle Transformation

Nellie was struggling with chronic pain, excess weight, and high blood sugar when she decided to turn her life around. While she knew she would achieve positive results, she didn't expect to recover a great, pain-free quality of life. In only a few months, Fascial Stretch Therapy helped her with weight loss, reduced her blood sugar levels, regulated her blood pressure, and dramatically improved her overall mental and physical well-being. Stretching has allowed her to adopt a healthy lifestyle. She replaced her unwanted addiction with a love for FST and fitness in general. Her favorite thing about stretching is that she walks away feeling rejuvenated and energized every time.

Emma's Cracked Disk Recovery

Emma had suffered from the consequences of a really bad fall, which resulted in a cracked disc in her spine. For 3 years, until she discovered the transformative power of stretching, she experienced severe pain. Moving around required a lot of strength, and walking was extremely painful for her. Shortly after the accident, Emma was diagnosed with osteoporosis and was prescribed medication and a specialized exercise plan. She hasn't stopped stretching ever since she first tried it 10 years ago. She went from thinking that she would live the rest of her life restricted and in pain to regaining mobility and experiencing an increase in her range of motion. She also mentioned that her bone density was up by 21% only one year after she implemented a stretch routine.

Steven's Life-Changing Stretching Experience

Steven struggles with osteoarthritis, which mostly impacts his hips and restricts his movements. He worked with a professional who considered his joints, bones, connective tissues, and muscles' conditions to devise a stretching routine tailored to his needs. In only a few months, the life-altering pain became manageable, and he gained strength in his hip muscles and mobility in his hip joints. He was surprised by how much easier it became for him to move and perform daily activities.

Walter's Enhanced Golf and Exercise Skills

Several areas of Walter's life significantly improved after he started stretching. He noticed that his golf skills became significantly better, his walking was quicker and more balanced, and all other forms of exercise were improved. His personal trainer at the gym even commented on how big a difference his stretch routine had made. He was mostly surprised by how strong his legs felt even after completing a standard 18-hole golf course. Walter stretches every morning and can easily notice the difference on days he doesn't.

Ruth's Pain-Free Life Experience at 78

Ruth was 75 years old when she experienced severe pain in the arch of her foot. While her orthopedic surgeon recommended surgery, explaining that it was the only way to relieve her pain, her son-in-law was adamant about having her try alternative methods. He contacted a doctor who diagnosed Ruth with mid-foot arthritis and recommended a certain stretch routine. Skeptical but willing to do anything to feel better, Ruth decided to give it a go. After 3 years of doing her stretch routine every day, she felt pain-free. At 78 years old, she was moving around better than she had in years.

Generations of Stretching Successes

Jenna decided to get her entire family started on stretching, claiming that it transformed life for herself, her mother, and her daughter.

Jenna's Increased Mobility and Flexibility

When she was younger, Jenna was generally active and flexible. However, life's obligations came in the way, which caused her to take on a more sedentary lifestyle. The less she moved, the more she felt stiff and in pain. Jenna also developed unbearable neck pain, for which her doctor recommended steroid shots. However, she knew that this was only a temporary fix. During her search for alternative solutions, she stumbled across the benefits of stretching.

Shortly after she gave it a try, Jenna was surprised to find that she regained mobility in her neck and shoulders and other areas in her body that she had never even realized were affected. Following a stretching routine opened Jenna's eyes to all the negative habits, like slouching and maintaining a bad posture, she had engaged in. She took corrective action and became more flexible than her teenage daughter.

Mia's Enhanced Posture and Increased Confidence

Jenna introduced her daughter, Mia, to her stretching regimen because Mia had a slouching problem. She had suddenly grown a lot taller than her friends, which made her feel insecure, causing her to slouch in an effort to appear shorter than she was. Additionally, Mia was never an active or flexible child, which added to her lack of self-confidence. She had always wanted to join the cheerleading team at school but was afraid to apply.

Jenna encouraged Mia to start stretching, and she eventually experienced improvements in her flexibility and self-confidence. She embraced her height and learned about the amazing things her body could do. Moreover, she made it into the cheerleading team. She went from hiding to becoming the team captain during her senior year of high school.

Alice's Pain Management

Lastly, Jenna's mother, Alice, struggled with osteoarthritis and rheumatoid arthritis. She felt excruciating pain in her knee to the point where the family thought she had torn her anterior cruciate ligament. Alice worked with a professional and determined that her tight hamstrings and hips were the main reasons behind her limited range of motion. They worked together to develop a stretching plan that suited Alice's needs and state, which proved very effective. Alice was astounded to find that she didn't need drugs to manage her pain. Only a few simple moves were needed to help her feel at ease.

Jenna always tells the story of how stretching has helped 3 generations of amazing women in her family and recommends it to everyone she meets.

Dr. Nina's Bounce Back from Ankle Replacement Surgery

Dr. Nina has been working as a physician for over 2 decades. According to her beliefs, physical exercises can benefit patients with musculoskeletal problems much more than any drugs could. So, when she developed back aches, Nina followed the same philosophy. She created a stretching regimen that was helpful in alleviating her pain. She later fractured her ankle and developed arthritis as a result. Even after her ankle replacement surgery, Nina was adamant about using stretching to manage her pain and regain her range of motion.

Eleanor's Stretching Journey at 93

Eleanor's son, Matt, decided to start a stretching program 2 years ago. She was astounded by his progress. Matt's endurance, fitness, and energy were a lot higher. It took her some convincing, but Eleanor finally decided to join Matt at the age of 93. She genuinely thought she was too old to feel any difference but told herself that it wouldn't hurt to try. Eleanor couldn't believe how good she felt. She ended up losing a lot of weight and gained mobility in her arms and thighs. She was elated when she discovered she could make her bed and do the dishes again.

Eva's Relief after Mastectomy

After having a mastectomy, Eva experienced a lot of tightness near her chest. She also had a decreased range of motion. She worked with a professional to develop a stretching plan that aligned with her treatment process. She felt much better after implementing her stretch routine and went home feeling very relaxed after every session.

Karen's Life-Changing Increase in Mobility

Karen was surprised at the life-changing enhancement in her physical capabilities and overall quality of life, which she achieved without medication. She started stretching 6 months after she was diagnosed with tennis elbow and plantar fasciitis. Karen thought she looked like a 50-year-old with the body of a 90-year-old. She struggled with shortened calf muscles and the permanent high-heeled position of her foot because she spent her entire youth wearing heels. A few months into stretching, Karen felt entirely pain-free. She went from struggling to touch her knees while bending to touching the floor with her hands. She has never felt more motivated to work on improving the rest of her body and building her strength, fitness, and endurance.

Daniel's Budokon Practice Achievement

Determined to support his sport and achieve his Budokon (a form of yoga) goals, Daniel decided to give stretching a try. Sitting on the heels is a necessary action in several Budokon movements. However, Daniel never seemed to get it right. He thought it was impossible to achieve the correct stance, but he discovered stretching just as he was starting to give up. He owes his success and his advancement in Budokon to Sylvia, his friend, who introduced him to his stretch routine.

Jennifer's Law Enforcement Career

Jennifer thought that her dreams of graduating from the police academy were lost when she was diagnosed with heel spurs, plantar fasciitis, and early shin splints. Walking, let alone running, was becoming an insurmountable challenge for her. Jennifer did everything she could think of, from investing in comfortable, medical-grade shoes to getting fancy, expensive massages.

She even tried various injections recommended by her doctors, but nothing she tried achieved positive results. She almost flunked the final physical section of her police training program but then she stumbled across a stretch training center. She worked with a professional almost every day until she recovered. Not only was Jennifer able to graduate, but she also felt the best she had in years. She believes she owes her career to the incredible power of stretching.

Joanna's Diminished Back and Neck Pains

Less than a year ago, Joanna struggled with relentless back and neck aches. Her medications weren't of much help, so she decided to take another route. After a lot of research, Joanna put a stretching routine together. She asked a professional to help her modify her plan and tailor it to her conditions. Joanna started stretching daily and supported her plan with a few other light exercises. She has gone from living in constant discomfort to being entirely pain-free. She says that she feels herself becoming more flexible and energized with each stretch. Joanna sings her praises to her stretching regimen to everyone she meets.

Maria and John's Transformative Discovery

Maria and John embarked on their stretch therapy journey together, reaching new heights in their path to wellness. The couple was surprised to learn that stretching was the missing link for which they had been searching for years. Their lower back and hip pains were no longer a problem, and they now enjoy an increased range of motion. Maria and John, who have been lifelong fitness companions, are now able to enjoy a plethora of fun and effective exercise routines. Their decreased pain levels allow them to go on adventures they never deemed possible in their 60s. Stretching was the reason behind their newfound vitality and strengthened relationship.

Conclusion

Stretching is a fun exercise you can practice at home. It doesn't require heavy equipment or daily trips to the gym. Children, adults, and senior citizens can perform this workout since it includes a variety of techniques suitable for all ages. It isn't an exaggeration to say that this form of exercise can change your life, and this book puts you on the right track.

This book starts by introducing stretching and its different types. It also sheds light on its significance and its effect on senior citizens and the process of aging.

You can't start stretching right away, especially if you are a beginner, or you risk injury. The book includes multiple warm-up exercises to prepare you mentally and physically before stretching. There are other things you should consider, too, like setting up a space at home for stretching and buying the necessary equipment. All this information was covered, including how to make your space warm and inviting.

Different stretches target every part of the body. The book provided various techniques with step-by-step instructions for these stretches. It also included full-body exercises, like tai chi and yoga stretches.

Some people think you should rest and avoid physical activities when you have a chronic condition. However, the reverse is true. Exercising can be effective in managing different symptoms. This book has offered various stretching techniques for specific conditions to reduce pain and make your life easier.

As you start stretching, you will notice physical changes, such as increased flexibility, and mental changes. You will also face challenges. Some people get bored or frustrated when performing the same exercise routine every day. This book explains in detail how your physical health will improve with stretching. It has also provided solutions on how to overcome exercise plateaus that halt your progress.

Resistance bands can make stretching more effective and fun. They have many health benefits and can transform your exercise routine. The book has suggested different strategies on how to incorporate these bands into your stretching exercises.

Some people get hurt when exercising. But this shouldn't scare or discourage you. You should take the necessary precautions to stay safe. The book explains the common mistakes people make while exercising, how to prevent injury, and when to consult a doctor.

Although stretching can improve your physical and mental health and well-being, you should do other things, too, for a healthy lifestyle. This book has discussed the impact of nutrition on flexibility and why you should stay hydrated. It has also provided techniques to reduce stress.

The last section of the book focuses on success stories of senior citizens whose lives have changed thanks to stretching.

These stories are meant to motivate you and encourage you to believe that you will achieve your goals if you keep practicing.

References

10 easy Tai Chi exercises for seniors. (2023, March 15). California Mobility. https://californiamobility.com/10-easy-tai-chi-exercises-for-seniors/

10 stretches to help your wrists and hands. (2014, July 14). Healthline. https://www.healthline.com/health/chronic-pain/wrist-and-hand-stretches

10 tips to eating healthy for older adults. (n.d.). Premierhealth.com. https://www.premierhealth.com/your-health/articles/women-wisdom-wellness-/10-tips-to-eating-healthy-for-older-adults

3 Ways to Increase Flexibility as You Age. (2022, June 5). Northwest Regional Health. https://northwestrh.org/3-ways-to-increase-flexibility-as-you-age/

5 Back and Neck Stretches to Do Every Day. (n.d.). Hss.edu. https://www.hss.edu/article_back-neck-stretches.asp

5 exercises to help ease chronic pain. (n.d.). Painscale.com. https://www.painscale.com/article/5-exercises-to-help-ease-chronic-pain

7 Stretching Mistakes and How to Avoid Them. (2019, January 8). Cary Orthopaedics. https://www.caryortho.com/7-stretching-mistakes-and-how-to-avoid-them/

8 tips for healthy eating. (n.d.). Nhs.uk. https://www.nhs.uk/live-well/eat-well/how-to-eat-a-balanced-diet/eight-tips-for-healthy-eating/

9 easy resistance band exercises for seniors. (2018, August 28). Camino Retirement Apartments; Lisa Witt. https://caminoretirement.com/2018/08/28/9-easy-resistance-band-exercises-for-seniors/

Admin, N. (2020, July 16). Safety Considerations for Exercising Older Adults. https://nsga.com/safety-considerations-for-exercising-older-adults/

Are, W. we. (n.d.). Simple and easy exercises for older adults. Age UK. https://www.ageuk.org.uk/information-advice/health-wellbeing/exercise/simple-exercises-inactive-adults/

Asp, K., MA, CPT, & VLCE. (n.d.). How You Stretch Matters—Avoid These 7 Common Mistakes to Stay Limber and Injury-Free. Real Simple. https://www.realsimple.com/health/fitness-exercise/stretching-yoga/streching-mistakes

Bedosky, L., & Rdn, R. F. M. (n.d.). Warm-up exercise: What it is, health benefits, and how to get started. Everydayhealth.com. https://www.everydayhealth.com/fitness/warm-up-exercises/guide/

Best hamstrings stretch routine for seniors. (n.d.). More Life Health - Seniors Health & Fitness. https://morelifehealth.com/hamstring-stretch

Best stretches for arthritis morning stiffness. (n.d.). WebMD. https://www.webmd.com/osteoarthritis/best-stretches

Biswas, C. (2021, November 29). 11 best stretching exercises for seniors (with pictures). STYLECRAZE. https://www.stylecraze.com/articles/stretching-exercises-for-seniors/

Bok, S.-K., Lee, T. H., & Lee, S. S. (2013). The effects of changes of ankle strength and range of motion according to aging on balance. Annals of Rehabilitation Medicine, 37(1), 10. https://doi.org/10.5535/arm.2013.37.1.10

Burgess, L. (2019, March 8). Top 10 shoulder stretches for pain and tightness. Medicalnewstoday.com. https://www.medicalnewstoday.com/articles/324647

Cadman, B. (2018, February 19). 9 foot exercises: For strengthening, flexibility, and pain relief. Medicalnewstoday.com. https://www.medicalnewstoday.com/articles/320964

Calf stretch. (2023, March 6). Mayo Clinic. https://www.mayoclinic.org/diseases-conditions/muscle-cramp/multimedia/calf-stretch/img-20007902

Chen, L. (2020, December 8). How to successfully overcome a workout plateau. Byrdie. https://www.byrdie.com/workout-plateau-5090487

Chronic pain. (n.d.). Cleveland Clinic. https://my.clevelandclinic.org/health/diseases/4798-chronic-pain

Chrysafidis, N. (2015, June 25). The 9 benefits of warm-up: Unleashing your full potential. Vertical Wise. https://www.verticalwise.com/warm-up/

Client Testimonials | StretchRx. (n.d.). https://stretchrxflorida.com/client-testimonials/

Constance Schein, R. N. (n.d.). The importance of staying hydrated. Aegisliving.com. https://www.aegisliving.com/resource-center/the-importance-of-staying-hydrated/

Cronkleton, E. (2017, April 26). How to increase stamina. Healthline. https://www.healthline.com/health/fitness-exercise/how-to-increase-stamina

Cronkleton, E. (2019, June 24). Bicep stretch: 6 stretches for upper arm strength. Healthline. https://www.healthline.com/health/bicep-stretch

Cronkleton, E. (2020, March 30). Passive stretching: Benefits, examples, and more. Healthline. https://www.healthline.com/health/exercise-fitness/passive-stretching

Cronkleton, E. (2022, April 29). 6 ways to bust through a workout plateau. Healthline. https://www.healthline.com/nutrition/workout-plateau

Effective exercises for osteoporosis. (2021, April 11). Harvard Health. https://www.health.harvard.edu/pain/effective-exercises-for-osteoporosis

Exercising With Chronic Conditions. (n.d.). National Institute on Aging. https://www.nia.nih.gov/health/exercising-chronic-conditions

familydoctor.org editorial staff, Rice, A., & familydoctor.org editorial staff, Alex Rice. (2017, July 26). Exercise and Seniors. Familydoctor.Org. https://familydoctor.org/exercise-seniors/

familydoctor.org editorial staff. (2004, September 1). Healthy Habits At 60 And Beyond - Diet And Exercise. Familydoctor.Org. https://familydoctor.org/healthy-habits-at-age-60-and-beyond/

Felman, A. (2023, September 29). Stretching exercises for seniors: Back, neck, and more. Medicalnewstoday.Com. https://www.medicalnewstoday.com/articles/stretching-exercises-for-seniors

Finberg, D. (2021). Health Benefits of Stretching for Older Adults. LifeSpanFitness. https://www.lifespanfitness.com/blogs/news/health-benefits-of-stretching-for-older-adults

Finlay, L. (2003, July 29). Here's how to choose the right resistance bands and how to use them. Verywell Fit. https://www.verywellfit.com/choosing-and-using-resistance-bands-1229709

Fitness Nation. (2019, October 29). How to break through your fitness plateau. Fitness Nation. https://fitness-nation.net/2019/10/29/how-to-break-through-your-fitness-plateau/

Fms/Sfma, O. a. D. S. M. C. C. M. U. (2020, April 20). Why Stretching and Maintaining Flexibility Can Slow Down Aging. . . LEVEL4 PT & Pilates. https://www.level4pt.com/flexibility-can-slow-down-aging/

Freutel, N. (2017, May 30). Exercises to reduce chronic pain. Healthline. https://www.healthline.com/health/exercises-to-reduce-chronic-pain

Get in the habit of stretching. (n.d.). Arthritis.org. https://www.arthritis.org/health-wellness/healthy-living/physical-activity/getting-started/get-in-the-habit-of-stretching

Gonzalez, J. C. (2021, September 14). 21 exercise equipment for seniors – how to choose the best one for your condition. Best Used Gym Equipment. https://www.bestusedgymequipment.com/exercise-equipment-for-seniors/

GoodRx - error. (n.d.). Goodrx.com. https://www.goodrx.com/well-being/movement-exercise/20-chair-exercises-for-seniors

Hall, T. (2023, March 23). 6 ways to avoid workout plateaus and keep your progress going strong. ASFA. https://www.americansportandfitness.com/blogs/fitness-blog/6-ways-to-avoid-workout-plateaus-and-keep-your-progress-going-strong

Healthy Bodies Physiotherapy. (2022). 7 Reasons Daily Stretches Are Important for People Over 60. Physiotherapy Services Cheltenham. https://www.healthybodiesphysiotherapy.com.au/7-reasons-daily-stretches-are-important-for-people-over-60/

Healthy meal planning: Tips for older adults. (n.d.). National Institute on Aging. https://www.nia.nih.gov/health/healthy-meal-planning-tips-older-adults

Hennessy, N. (2022, December 21). 10 hydration tips for seniors. IRT. https://www.irt.org.au/the-good-life/10-hydration-tips-for-seniors/

Hernández-Guillén, D., Tolsada-Velasco, C., Roig-Casasús, S., Costa-Moreno, E., Borja-de-Fuentes, I., & Blasco, J.-M. (2021). Association ankle function and balance in community-dwelling older adults. PloS One, 16(3), e0247885. https://doi.org/10.1371/journal.pone.0247885

Hip strengthening exercises for seniors. (n.d.). Onemedical.com. https://www.onemedical.com/blog/exercise-fitness/hip-strengthening-exercises-for-seniors/

How Older Adults Can Get Started With Exercise. (n.d.). National Institute on Aging. https://www.nia.nih.gov/health/how-older-adults-can-get-started-exercise

How to relieve stress: Breathing exercises you can do anywhere. (2021, March 30). The Jed Foundation. https://jedfoundation.org/resource/how-to-relieve-stress-breathing-exercises-you-can-do-anywhere/

How to set up the perfect space for stretching. (n.d.). Stretching Videos for Flexibility | STRETCHIT. https://stretchitapp.com/blog/stretching-space

Inverarity, L. (2005, July 11). 3 easy ways to stretch tight quads. Verywell Fit. https://www.verywellfit.com/quadricep-stretches-2696366

Judson Senior Living. (2016, April 4). 5 Ways Older Adults Can Reduce Stress. Judson. https://www.judsonsmartliving.org/blog/5-ways-older-adults-can-reduce-stress/

Kapoor, A. K. (1618637900000). Benefits of flexibility Exercises for Seniors: 12 important reasons. Linkedin.com. https://www.linkedin.com/pulse/benefits-flexibility-exercises-seniors-12-important-reasons-kapoor/

Lautieri, A. (2019, March 13). Visualization and guided imagery techniques for stress reduction. Mentalhelp.net; admin. https://www.mentalhelp.net/stress/visualization-and-guided-imagery-techniques-for-stress-reduction/

Loria, K. (2022, July 11). Staying flexible and healthy as you age. Washington Post. https://www.washingtonpost.com/health/2022/07/11/stretching-helps-aging-bodies/

Marcin, A. (2017, July 12). Ankle stretches: Strengthening, flexibility, and more. Healthline. https://www.healthline.com/health/fitness-exercise/ankle-stretches

Millar, H. (2020, October 5). Stretching routine: Daily full body stretches and more. Medicalnewstoday.com. https://www.medicalnewstoday.com/articles/stretching-routine

Miller, A. (2021, October 14). 3 common resistance band problems. Fabrication Enterprises; Fabrication Enterprises Inc. https://www.fab-ent.com/3-common-resistance-band-problems/

Neck pain. (2022, August 25). Mayo Clinic. https://www.mayoclinic.org/diseases-conditions/neck-pain/symptoms-causes/syc-20375581

No title. (n.d.). Anytimefitness.com. https://www.anytimefitness.com/ccc/how-to-break-through-a-workout-plateau/

Nunez, K. (2019, August 22). How to stretch glutes: 7 ways to ease tightness and tension. Healthline. https://www.healthline.com/health/exercise-fitness/how-to-stretch-glutes

Nutrition Secrets That Can Help Your Flexibility Training. (n.d.). Stretching Videos for Flexibility | STRETCHIT. https://stretchitapp.com/blog/nutrition-and-flexibility

Oerman, A. (2021, November 2). The 5 best arm stretches you can do basically anywhere. Cosmopolitan. https://www.cosmopolitan.com/health-fitness/a38036569/best-arm-stretches/

One Stretch. (2016, July 8). Real Stories - Testimonials - One Stretch. https://onestretch.com/testimonials/

Paige Waehner, C. P. T. (2016, January 15). Total Body Stretch for Seniors. Verywell Fit. https://www.verywellfit.com/total-body-stretch-for-seniors-1230960

Petersen, J. (2023, August 9). How long does it take to improve flexibility? Petersen Physical Therapy. https://petersenpt.com/how-long-does-it-take-to-improve-flexibility

Plantar fasciitis. (2021, August 8). Hopkinsmedicine.org. https://www.hopkinsmedicine.org/health/conditions-and-diseases/plantar-fasciitis

Polizzi, M. (2021, January 15). Hip Stretches for Seniors. Verywell Health. https://www.verywellhealth.com/hip-stretches-for-seniors-5095639

Precautions for Flexibility Activities. (n.d.). Healthlinkbc.Ca. https://www.healthlinkbc.ca/healthy-eating-physical-activity/being-active/injury-prevention-and-recovery/precautions

Rao, J. (2015, March 13). 5 best chair cardio exercises to burn calories. STYLECRAZE. https://www.stylecraze.com/articles/best-chair-cardio-exercises-to-burn-calories/

Reddy, R. S., & Alahmari, K. A. (2016). Effect of lower extremity stretching exercises on balance in geriatric population. International Journal of Health Sciences, 10(3), 389.

Roberts, J. (2019, June 16). 10 yoga poses for seniors. YOGA PRACTICE. https://yogapractice.com/yoga/10-yoga-poses-for-seniors/

Role of exercise in arthritis management. (2011, April 13). Johns Hopkins Arthritis Center. https://www.hopkinsarthritis.org/patient-corner/disease-management/role-of-exercise-in-arthritis-management/

Scott, E. (2006, May 16). How to practice basic meditation for stress management. Verywell well. https://www.verywellmind.com/practice-basic-meditation-for-stress-management-3144789

Seated hamstring muscule stretch for seniors. (n.d.). More Life Health - Seniors Health & Fitness. https://morelifehealth.com/seated-hamstring-stretch

Set, S. F. (2022). 13 best stretches for seniors that can be done standing or seated. SET FOR SET. https://www.setforset.com/blogs/news/stretches-for-seniors

Setting up your ultimate stretching space. (2021, August 23). WeStretch. https://westretch.ca/blog/setting-up-your-ultimate-stretching-space/

Simple Warmup. (n.d.). Simplewarmup.com. https://www.simplewarmup.com/

Solis-Navarro, L., Masot, O., Torres-Castro, R., Otto-Yáñez, M., Fernández-Jané, C., Solà-Madurell, M., Coda, A., Cyrus-Barker, E., Sitjà-Rabert, M., & Pérez, L. M. (2023). Effects on sleep quality of physical exercise programs in older adults: A systematic review and meta-analysis. Clocks & Sleep, 5(2), 152–166. https://doi.org/10.3390/clockssleep5020014

Stathokostas, L., D. Little, R. M., Vandervoort, A. A., & Paterson, D. H. (2012). Flexibility Training and Functional Ability in Older Adults: A Systematic Review. Journal of Aging Research, 2012. https://doi.org/10.1155/2012/306818

Stelter, G. (2014, August 14). 5 seated back pain stretches for seniors. Healthline. https://www.healthline.com/health/back-pain/stretches-for-seniors

Stew Smith, C. (2021, September 7). Why You Should Consult Your Doctor Before Starting an Exercise Program. Military.Com. https://www.military.com/military-fitness/why-you-should-consult-your-doctor-starting-exercise-program

Testimonials - Stretch Recovery Lounge | Assisted Stretching and Athletic Recovery Facility. (2022, March 30). Stretch Recovery Lounge | Assisted Stretching and Athletic Recovery Facility. https://stretchrecoverylounge.com/testimonials/

Testimonials - Stretching Your Life. (2023, February 23). Stretching Your Life. https://www.stretchingyourlife.com/testimonials/

Testimonials – Stretch Therapy Boston. (n.d.). http://stretchtherapyboston.org/testimonials/

Testimonials – StretchingSA. (n.d.). https://www.stretchingsa.co.za/testimonials-2/

Testimonials — Jo Stretch. (n.d.). Jo Stretch. https://www.jostretch.com/testimonials

Testimonials — Sandlen Stretch Therapy. (n.d.). Sandlen Stretch Therapy. https://www.sandlenstretchtherapy.com/testimonials-1

The Stretching InstituteTM. (2022, September 13). Testimonials, Endorsements & Reviews | StretchCoach.com. StretchCoach.com | Stretching and Flexibility. https://stretchcoach.com/products/testimonials/

Thomason, K., & Breitowich, A. (2019, February 27). 10 best warm-up exercises from trainers to start every workout strong. Women's Health. https://www.womenshealthmag.com/fitness/g26554730/best-warm-up-exercises/

Top 6 Steps to Manage Stress. (n.d.). @NCOAging. https://www.ncoa.org/article/stress-and-how-to-reduce-it-a-guide-for-older-adults

Topia, T. (2022, October 17). Warm-up exercises for seniors that stimulate relaxation and improve overall health. True Topia. https://truetopia.com/best-warm-up-exercises-for-seniors/

Types of Stretching. (2012, November 19). https://www.acefitness.org/fitness-certifications/ace-answers/exam-preparation-blog/2966/types-of-stretching/

Usa, H. (2022). Why Stretching is Important in Active Aging and Functional Training. HUR USA - FOR LIFELONG STRENGTH. https://hurusa.com/why-stretching-is-important-in-active-aging-and-functional-training/

Vive Health. (n.d.). 22 chair exercises for seniors & how to get started. Vive Health. https://www.vivehealth.com/blogs/resources/chair-exercises-for-seniors

Walker, B. (2001, November 23). What is a warm-up? Stretchcoach.com | Stretching and Flexibility; The Stretching InstituteTM. https://stretchcoach.com/articles/warm-up/

Winks), D. W. (dani. (2022, June 13). Not making progress stretching? 7 reasons why —. Dani Winks Flexibility. https://www.daniwinksflexibility.com/bendy-blog/not-making-progress-stretching-x-reasons-why

Printed in Dunstable, United Kingdom

65085095R00111